KEYS TO A HEALTHY SMILE AFTER 40

7 Secrets to Feeling 7 Years Younger

Drs. Justene and Janice Doan

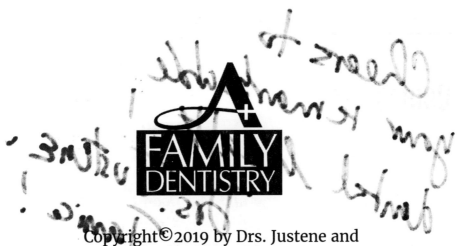

Copyright©2019 by Drs. Justene and
Janice Doan and Published by
A+ Family Dentistry
3780 El Cajon Blvd, Unit#1
San Diego, CA 92105

This book is of a general nature and does
not substitute for regular visits to your doctor and dentist. Please see your dentist every
three months for a cleaning, checkup, and
advice tailored specifically to your needs,
goals, and health.

ISBN: 978-1074537647

Dedication

To our parents Long and Mai Doan for your love, sacrifice, and wisdom which gave us our future and our freedom.

To our staff and patients for your love and support which allows us to do work that we love every day.

To Aurora Winter—without your help and guidance, this book would not have been possible.

Justene & Janice Doan

Contents

Preface

HOW THIS BOOK WILL HELP YOU

"Keys to a Healthy Smile After 40" shatters the myth that plastic surgery is the best way to rejuvenate your face. The truth is— the best way to rejuvenate your face is to have a healthy smile.

Most people have no clue that they can prevent disease and reverse aging through proper dental care. It's not their fault—no one has taken the time to explain the truth. Until now.

Dr. Justene Doan and Dr. Janice Doan reveal why you need different dental care after age 40. They share seven steps that will help you look and feel seven years younger. You can become healthier, more confident, and more attractive by following their proven system.

It's not too late to turn back the clock and regain a beautiful, youthful smile!

3

You will learn:

- Why bone loss jeopardizes your health, self-confidence and beauty

- How throat cancer can be detected in 3 minutes and save your life

- Why your smile gradually fades as you age, and what to do about it now

- The shocking connection between poor oral health and increased risk of heart attack or stroke

- The surprising link between your smile and your income

- Action steps you can take to regain your health and youthful vitality, starting today

- Why increases in life expectancy make dental care more important than ever

- And much more!

Dr. Justene Doan, DDS and Dr. Janice Doan, DDS understand dental care both personally and professionally. They both have beautiful, healthy white smiles today—but it wasn't always that way.

The Doan sisters were born in Vietnam. After the war, their prospects were bleak. The girls tried to escape but were captured and imprisoned in a concentration camp. They didn't have enough to eat—or even a toothbrush. Their teeth were full of cavities. This book reveals the miraculous story of their harrowing escape from Vietnam to America.

After receiving dental care in the US and experiencing first-hand the transformation in their health, confidence, and smiles, the Doan sisters decided to become dentists and founded A+ Family Dentistry in San Diego.

They now help others using their unique branded system of empathy, education, and the latest breakthrough techniques in dentistry. Patients travel for hours to experience their unique brand of caring dentistry. Other dentists benefit from their transformative training. To find out how they can help you, too, visit: www.APlusFamilyDentistry.com.

Introduction

Aurora:

I'm Aurora Winter, TV writer-producer, author, and interviewer. The backbone of this book is a wide-ranging interview with my amazing clients and friends, Drs. Justene and Janice Doan, founders of A+ Family Dentistry.

Our conversation covers the keys to a healthy smile after the age of 40 and 7 secrets to feeling 7 years younger. This book is an easy read in a conversational style, yet we are going on quite the journey.

You will learn how to reverse the signs of aging so that you can look and feel younger and healthier. You will learn the shocking link between poor oral health and an increased risk of heart attack or stroke. You'll also learn the surprising connection between your smile, your self-confidence, and your income.

Also—for the first time—the Doan sisters will share their harrowing escape from Vietnam to America in the aftermath of the Vietnam War, including their imprisonment in a concentration camp. In spite of those challenges—or perhaps because of them—they are two of the most positive people that I know.

I hope you enjoy this book and this interview with Janice and Justene Doan as much as I did. Let's get started.

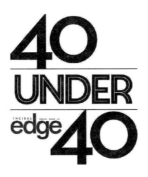

Top 40 Under 40

Aurora:

Welcome, Justene and Janice. Most people know you as experts, as caring, professional dentists. Yet there is a lot more to both of you!

Yesterday, I visited A+ Family Dentistry in San Diego, California. I love the fact that you have massage chairs. Every dentist should have massage chairs! You're ahead of the curve with innovations that make a visit to the dentist more comfortable. And you have all the latest equipment so that you can deliver precise, accurate, high-quality dental care.

I noticed photos on your waiting room wall celebrating that you were both celebrated as the "Top 40 Under 40" in the magazine "Incisal Edge." That's quite the honor. How did that happen?

Justene:

Benco Dental is one of the largest dental supply companies in the US. Their representatives travel around to different dental offices. When they came to our office, they saw that we have very up-to-date, modern technology. They saw the quality of care and procedures that we deliver to our patients. So they were impressed.

Aurora:

I'm not surprised. I was impressed when I went to your offices yesterday. You have seven chairs and latest equipment.

Recently I visited another dentist in another city because my crown fell off. They're a well-known, reputable dentist with a large office, but you two are head and shoulders above what they're doing.

Some things stood out to me at A+ Family Dentistry. I appreciated the warm, personal welcome, the tour of your facilities, taking a photograph of each patient's face, and taking the time to connect with each patient. I loved your massage chairs.

The other thing I found helpful was that, in addition to dental X-rays, you also take actual photographs, so that the patient can see their real teeth. Dentists are used to reading X-rays, but for patients, it's much more clear and understandable to see photographs of their teeth and inside their mouth.

And you are keeping up with the latest technology and investing in the latest new technology. When you gave me the tour of A+ Family Dentistry, you showed me some brand new equipment.

Justene:
Yes, we just got a cone beam CT scan.

Aurora:
What does that do?

Justene:
Three-dimensional imaging. X-rays show only two dimensions. For example, X-rays show height and width, but not thickness. So the cone beam CT scan allows us to view

the jaw in three dimensions. So we have very accurate information. As a result, I noticed an improvement in my diagnosing and delivering of dentistry.

Aurora:

Of course, because then you have the data right there, visually, in front of you.

Janice:

Yes.

Aurora:

What happened that resulted in you both being acknowledged as in the top 40 dentists under 40 in the United States?

Justene:

The representatives of Benco Dental saw our patients and our approach. Our office is different than other dental offices. For example, our patients are a lot more engaged.

Typically, in other dental offices, the doctor talks a lot, and at some point, the patient glazes over and is not participating. In contrast, at our offices, patients are asking questions, patients are engaged, so they saw that difference.

As a result, we were nominated for top 40 under 40 in 2015.

Janice:
And we won!

Aurora:
Congratulations! So you two are in the top 40 dentists under 40 in the nation.

Justene:
I'm over 40 now, so I'm both personally and professionally aware of the issues confronting people over 40.

Aurora:
Yesterday, you walked me through your unique branded system for welcoming new patients. So many little details added up to make a big impression.

One of the first things, was when you were showing me the room where the dental chair is, there was a little chalkboard that said, "Welcome, Aurora," with a big smiley face. You always do that with your patients. You welcome people, put them at ease, communicate how much you care.

Justene:

We do care.

Aurora:

I'm sure that contributed to you winning the top 40 under 40. Janice, you look great in this magazine. That's quite the stunning scarlet gown you're wearing at the awards ceremony.

Janice:

Thank you, I had just had my baby in June of 2014, and then when they nominated us, and we got selected, it was beginning of 2015. That was six months after I had delivered, so I didn't have my figure back yet. But I decided to go to the awards ceremony. Once I got there, they had many different dresses, jewelry, and shoes.

Aurora:

You look stunning—dressed as if for the Oscars.

Janice:

Thank you.

Aurora:

"Friendly Dentistry" magazine has also featured you in an article. You two are popular with the media. Congratulations.

Later, we're going to cover the things that people absolutely must know to enjoy healthy teeth and gums and a beautiful, brilliant smile at every age.

But first, and I'd love you to share your personal story. Where were you born? What was your childhood like?

Challenging Beginnings

Justene:
Both Janice and I were born in Vietnam. I was born in 1975, right after the Vietnam War. Luckily, I still remember a lot of my childhood. It was difficult, it was struggle, but I don't think of it as bad, you know?

I think because of my childhood, I value having the opportunity to help people a lot more. So my childhood was difficult. My father was in a concentration camp.

The Vietnam War was over in April 1975, and I was born in June. Immediately after April, my dad was incarcerated in a concentration camp.

For the first two years of my life, my poor mom didn't know where he was. I remember traveling on bus with her, looking for my dad. So that was a little tough.

Aurora:
A little tough? That's an understatement!

Justene:

I remember my mom was very distressed and worried at the time, not knowing where my dad was.

Aurora:

Of course.

Justene:

I didn't understand all of that at the time, but I could feel my mom's emotions. She was worried and distressed.

Aurora:

That must have given you a lot of empathy.

Justene:

I think so. I think that allowed me to see patients with more empathy and insight. These days, at times I sense what others are feeling. It's not the words my patients say; it's more of a vibration. An emotion that I can intuitively feel.

Aurora:

You sense their worry, their concern, their uncertainty?

Justene:

It's never spoken. It's something that you feel, but it's not spoken.

Aurora:

You're intuitive because of that experience as a child.

So, when did you mother find your father in the concentration camp?

Justene:

I think after a year, year and a half.

Aurora:

A year and a half of searching? Wow!

Justene:

Yes. Once my mother found where our father was being held, we visited him every two or three months. The concentration camp was far away from our home, and we were very poor at the time, so we would have to travel by bus. After the war, the country was really poor. We were poor.

Aurora:

Who was holding him in the concentration camp if the war was over?

Justene:
My dad was in the South Vietnam army. Vietnam was in civil war, the North and the South were fighting. The North won, so basically, the government was holding South Vietnamese soldiers, including my dad, in concentration camps.

Aurora:
What were the conditions in the concentration camp?

Justene:
Food was in very short supply. Prisoners were forced to do manual labor. They lived in little huts. Later, I asked my dad about it, but he doesn't want to talk about it much.

Aurora:
I can respect that. He doesn't want to go back there, right?

Justene:
Yes, it was not a good time for him.

Aurora:
Were you alive then, Janice?

Janice:

I wasn't. I was born in 1981, and he was out by then.

Afterward, I was curious, and I asked my dad about it. He was young at that time—in his early 20s—when he was in the concentration camp.

Justene:

After our dad was released from the concentration camp, he wasn't allowed to be in a big city. The government was afraid that the former soldiers from the South Vietnamese army would get together and rebel. So they were forced to spread out in rural areas.

Aurora:

What do you remember about when your father was released? What happened?

Justene:

When he was released, he was asked to relocate to his hometown [Nha Trang], which is in a rural area. I remember when he got out, my mom was thrilled!

But then after that, mom and dad moved to that small town, and I was left behind. I stayed with my grandparents in the big city of Saigon [Ho Chi Minh]. So I didn't grow up with my parents at all.

Forced to live in a small town, the Doans decided to send their daughters to Saigon to have a better education and the chance for a better life.

Aurora:
Oh, that's a surprise. How did you feel about that?

Justene:
My grandparents were very loving, and they explained to me that I needed to go to school, to get better opportunities. And the education was much better in the city.

Aurora:
That makes sense.

Justene:
I grew up with my grandparents, who are a lot older. Sometimes I questioned why my parents weren't with me.

But at that time it wasn't a big problem because emotions were secondary to basic survival. Having food, water, shelter, and education were the priorities.

Aurora:

Was it dangerous for you to join your parents in their hometown?

Justene:

I don't think it was dangerous, but I appreciate the education that I got in the city of Saigon. In Nha Trang, the small town where my parents lived, a good education was not available.

Janice:

There was no school there.

Aurora:

That's one of the things I'm passionate about—education. Education is the key to a better future.

Justene:

Right.

Aurora:

As a little aside, when I was about 14 years old, we lived in Indonesia for a while. My father was the head of a Canadian International Development Agency (CIDA) project that had the mission of helping Indonesians have a better, healthier life with more abundant food. Families on this CIDA project lived in a cluster of houses.

There was a village right beside us, and the village chief was suffering from malaria. The water in their well was infected with mosquitoes that cause malaria. We didn't have showers with hot running water. Instead, there was an open storage tank with room temperature water in the corner of the bathroom. We dipped into that water to wash. Mosquito larva swam in that water.

I had never thought about how precious clean water is before that. Realizing how blessed I am, changed my life in a profound and valuable way.

I was surprised to have more culture shock coming back from Indonesia than going there. I came back to North America, and we're all driving on these beautifully paved four-lane highways, we have cars not bicycles, we're not on foot. We have—not bare feet—but so many different kinds of shoes. In Indonesia, you're rich if you have a bicycle. You're rich if you have a pair of running shoes.

But when you turn on the news in North America, it's filled with bad news. People are complaining that they don't have enough money, times are tough. It was shocking to me. People living in North America are so lucky, but so unaware of their good fortune.

Justene:

Totally.

Aurora:

Living in Indonesia changed my life in a good way. I became more grateful. I gained a broader perspective.

For you, was it life-changing to come from Vietnam to America?

Justene:

Totally. And I wouldn't have it any other way. I appreciate living here very, very much.

In Vietnam, I remember getting in line to get rice. And the rice was so bad. It was non-edible! At two or three years old, I sat and separated the edible from the non-edible when I was in Vietnam.

Aurora:

Not many two-year-olds have to do that. That reminds me of Viktor Frankl's book "Man's Search For Meaning."

It's a profound book about his experience in a concentration camp. He shares noticing bugs in his rice and choosing to eat them for the protein because he was at death's door. They were fed so little in the concentration camp.

How did you escape?

Escaping Vietnam

Justene:

Our first attempt to escape Vietnam was in 1983. Janice was one, and our brother was a baby, just a few months old. We escaped by boat.

My dad didn't go with us. The risk was too high. If he got caught, he could face the death sentence.

So it was just my mom and the three kids.

WE ESCAPED BY BOAT IN THE DEAD OF NIGHT

Our parents were worried about our future. They wanted us to have a better life, better education, better future. Even though I was going to grade school, my opportunities would be restricted because of my dad's background in the South Vietnamese army.

Also, when I turn 18, I would have to go into army. Vietnam was constantly at war with the Chinese at the time. My parents didn't want me to be in the army.

Aurora:

So there were a lot of reasons to escape, in spite of the risk.

Justene:

We escaped at night. I wasn't informed what was going to happen. I just followed along.

We went to the beach at night, which was weird. It was pitch dark, and we were with a bunch of strangers. My uncle, my mom's brother, went with us.

I was eight years old. They put me in this basket with two strangers, both men, and they were paddling out to a big boat.

I didn't know how to swim. I didn't know the men in the basket. I didn't know what's going on.

I was told to be quiet by mom. My mom went a different way, so I was separated from my family. I was quiet.

We arrived at a big boat. It was completely dark. We didn't want to get caught, so there was no light.

I had the sense that there were about a hundred people in the boat.

I got onto the boat from the basket, and it took a couple hours for me to find my uncle; it was so dark.

Aurora:
You must have been frightened, as an eight-year-old alone on a dark boat with a hundred strangers.

Justene:
When I found there my uncle, he told me, "Your mom is on the boat. Don't worry. You stay with me."

I didn't see my mom and my brother and sister until the next day. I spent the night with my uncle and a lot of other people in the boat.

Aurora:
Were you able to lay down and sleep?

Justene:

No, it was more like sitting. It was tight. My uncle sat up most of the night. I was able to curl up for a bit, but it was cramped quarters.

Aurora:

Did you have anything with you besides your clothes?

Justene:

Just my clothes. I think my mom brought some things, but I didn't carry anything with me.

Aurora:

You must have been terrified.

Justene:

It was an adventure.

Aurora:

I love your positive attitude! An adventure, okay.

Justene:

I mean, I was on high alert. So many things were happening, it was a lot to take in.

The good thing about being a kid, is sometimes you're not so scared, you know? I had a heightened feeling, but I don't remember being terrified.

Aurora:

Well, your uncle and your mom did a good job of, "Let's go on an adventure!"

That's how my mom always was when we traveled as kids, "Let's go on an adventure!"

I bought it, "Okay!" It's a great attitude to go through life, isn't it?

So then what happened?

Justene:

I found my sister and my brother and my mom the next day. We were out on the ocean for three nights and four days. We had little to eat. Going to the bathroom was a little scary.

Aurora:

How did you go to the bathroom?

Justene:

I remember they had these little buckets, and it was kind of gross. There were about a hundred people on the boat. It was a very basic boat. There was no toilet.

Aurora:
A fishing boat, probably?

Justene:
Yes, it was probably a fishing boat.

Aurora:
Probably suited to 12 people, not 100.

Justene:
Yes, so I remember I would try not to go to the bathroom.

Aurora:
Right, and then you really have to go.

Justene:
Then I'd have to go. We were on the lower deck. People were whispering, we were trying to be quiet.

And then, on the fourth morning, after three nights, the fourth morning, I heard a commotion on the deck. Adults were reacting with fear, worry, anger. I could feel the different emotions in the adults around me.

Aurora:

You're perceptive.

Justene:

Yes. I could feel the change in the emotion. Even though people were quiet, there was a lot of noise on the upper deck. We got caught.

Aurora:

Oh, no!

Justene:

So the boat had to turn around.

Aurora:

Who caught you?

Justene:

The Vietnamese military. We still hadn't left Vietnam. So the escape failed, and the boat was turned around.

It took a few hours and we were once again on a beach. But it was a different beach, and we were getting off the boat this time. Then we went into a concentration camp.

Aurora:

Oh, no! So you didn't go back to where you started. You were taken to a concentration camp?

Janice:

We were taken to a concentration camp.

Justene:

Right.

Aurora:

Wow. An eight-year-old in a concentration camp. And Janice was how old?

Janice:

I was one. One and a half.

Justene:

And our brother was a baby—just a few months old. Mom was breastfeeding him.

Aurora:

So your mother was put in the concentration camp with a baby, a toddler, and an eight-year-old. Oh, my goodness. And your uncle?

Janice:

Him, too.

Aurora:

He wasn't shot. That's a relief.

What was the concentration camp like?

Justene:

Well, it was very crowded. Huts in the middle of a small town near the beach. Each day we had to get in line to take a shower, and get water. They gave us instant rice. I remember the rice, I don't remember any protein or vegetables to go along with it. We were there for a month.

Aurora:

Do you remember arriving at the concentration camp?

Justene:

I remember getting off the boat. I'm not sure what has happened.

And then I heard fragments of what the adults were saying, things like, "We didn't make it," or, "We're turning around, hope things are going to be okay."

Aurora:

Right. And were you still feeling it was an adventure? Or were you terrified?

Justene:

Well, I was worried at that time.

Aurora:

I can see how this experience would give you empathy. Give you the capacity to be caring and compassionate for other people when they're dealing with adversity.

Janice:

She does have a lot of empathy.

Aurora:

What stands out to you from that time, Janice? What is your first memory as a child?

Janice:

I do remember going in the forest and going to the beach and getting on the boat. A lot a people running, and I didn't know what's going on. I was sleeping, there were a lot of noises, and it was just hectic. Even though everyone was trying to be quiet, I could still hear a lot of noises. But I was too young, so I didn't comprehend what was going on.

I don't remember seeing my sister or my uncle. I just remember my mom and my baby brother. My mom was holding my brother, and I'm trying to stay close to her, so I don't get lost because there were so many people.

Aurora:

Easy to get separated in a crowd of people in the dark.

Janice:

Yes.

Aurora:

And strange circumstances.

Janice:

Yes.

Aurora:

When you were in the concentration camp, did you only eat rice?

Janice:

I was only one, so I was still being breastfed. My mom fed my baby brother first, then me.

Aurora:

You were getting scraps!

Janice:

Yeah, after my brother's done, then it's my turn.

Aurora:

And your mother is surviving on instant rice.

Janice:

Yes.

Aurora:

Did people die?

Janice:

I'm sure. I saw people get really skinny, really sick, coughing, really dirty.

Aurora:

What was your most powerful memory from that time?

Janice:

Seeing other people around me doing nothing, and not being able to do anything about our condition. Feeling helpless.

Aurora:

That's a horrible feeling. Helpless.

Janice:

Yes. No one wants to be there. But we're being forced to stay.

Aurora:

One of the things that I've noticed about you, Janice, is that you're so bubbly, so happy, so optimistic. You always have this huge, dazzling smile. I don't think I've met any-one else who is so cheerful and enthusiastic.

Janice:

Thanks.

Aurora:

Do you think that that came from the con-trast of knowing hard times? So that you feel more grateful today? How do you think adversity as a child formed your personality as an adult?

Janice:

When I was younger, a lot of times I was not allowed to be part of the decision mak-ing. People dismissed me, like, "Oh, you're just a kid, you don't know what's going on."

As a kid, you're not allowed to know what's happening. You're just expected to follow what the adults are doing. If you want to do something else, you're not allowed. There's no choice, no information, no options.

Aurora:

I can see that might be why you care so much to let people understand what you're doing in your profession now as a dentist. It's important to you that your patients know what their choices are and have freedom of choice.

Janice:

Exactly.

Aurora:

I notice that you take a lot of time with your patients, and really help them make choices. They have the information. You show them photographs of their teeth and X-rays. You explain the short-term and long-term consequences of proper dental care. You make it clear with diagrams and photographs. That really stood out to me yesterday at your office.

Janice:

Absolutely. I think that's one of the things that formed me as a child. Today, doing dentistry, I want other people to know what's going on and have that ability to say, "This is what I want to do to improve my condition," or, "No, I don't want to do it this way, because blah blah blah."

I never want my patients to feel that they are being treated like a child. I want them to be empowered to make wise, informed decisions as an adult.

Growing up, I had the privilege of staying with our grandparents who took excellent care of me. Seeing myself compared to the other kids in our neighborhood who were less fortunate, made me feel grateful of what I had, even though we didn't have much.

Aurora:

It's all relative. What did your grandparents do that made them a little more affluent than the others in the neighborhood?

Janice:

From what I remember, my grandpa was working part-time, but my grandma was not working. She moved from North Vietnam down to South Vietnam. My grandma used to be a teacher, but she was no longer working by the time I was there. She was mainly taking care of me and my sister, and then my brother a year later.

But luckily we have an aunt who is my mom's younger sister, who escaped before the war. My aunt got to France, and she was able to make money over there and send us money.

So I don't think it's because our family worked more, or were more affluent. We were just able to get someone to help us financially, from a foreign country.

Justene:

My grandmother was a great woman. She knew how to run the household. Back in Vietnam, you have to have one person to run the household.

We didn't have a refrigerator, so she would have to go and get groceries every single day. I remember going to the grocery store with her. She would bargain for good food at a better price.

My aunt in France was sending money home. Other people would want to send money to a relative, and my grandmother would facilitate that, and she would get a commission.

My grandmother is 92 years old this year. This is my maternal grandmother. She's still in Vietnam, and she's still doing the same thing. Mentally she's sharp, and she continues to count money and deliver money to other people.

She was a strong, capable woman. She was my first teacher. She taught me how to write the alphabet.

Aurora:

Great to have a teacher for a grandmother.

Justene:

Yes. I learned how to write alphabet at two or three years old.

Aurora:

You're a sponge for learning. You started early with your grandmother.

Is your aunt still alive? The one that was in France?

Janice:

Yes.

Aurora:

You have a caring, connected family.

Let's pick it up where we left off a moment ago. You were at the concentration camp, and you were eight years old, right?

Justene:
Right.

Aurora:
What happened after you arrived at the concentration camp?

Justene:
One of the most traumatic experiences there, was on the third night, as I recall.

IN THE MIDDLE OF THE NIGHT, I HEARD A GUNSHOT

In the middle of the night, I heard a gunshot.

Aurora:
A gunshot!

Justene:
Somebody tried to escape. Somehow, I always feel the energy of other people. I felt the fear. I felt the grief.

I heard a gunshot in the middle of the night, and then there were noises. My mom told me, "Go back to sleep."

The next day I heard the adult talking, "Somebody tried to escape and got shot last night." It was never confirmed. But I knew it had happened.

Aurora:

You sensed the energy. You're perceptive. Intuitive.

Justene:

Yes. I felt the energy.

Aurora:

Terror was broadcast energetically.

Justene:

Yes, it's definitely a form of communication. It's not verbal. It's a stronger form of communication for me at times.

Aurora:

Yes, I agree. I think we're like tuning forks, and we pick up the vibration of what's happening, especially nearby. Or we tune in to somebody far away that we love.

For example, when my mother had her stroke, I sensed it. I was the first one there, even though no one called me. But that's another story for another time.

Perhaps these traumatic events strengthened your intuitive abilities. Almost like learning a language. You learned the language of perception, of empathy, of intuition as a child.

Justene:

Yes, I think so. In Vietnamese culture, children are not allowed to speak much. That's what Janice was saying. We were told to be quiet, and only speak when spoken to.

Janice:

I'd get hit when I would try to say something. The adults didn't want to hear from me. I would get slapped a lot.

Aurora:

Really?

Janice:

Yes.

Aurora:

Wow.

(teasing)

Is this still happening?

Janice:

Well not now!

Aurora:

(smiling)

Just kidding, just kidding.

Janice:

(laughs)

I know my big sister is doing most of the talking right now. But there's no slapping!

Aurora:

That used to be common in our culture in North America, too. "Children should be seen and not heard."

So in Vietnam, it was normal to slap kids if they're too noisy?

Janice:

Right.

Aurora:

Did you experience that as physical abuse? Or did you just experience that as you didn't have the right to speak?

Janice:

Both. As a kid, getting hit is really painful.

Aurora:

True.

Janice:

Getting hit conditions kids not to speak up.

Aurora:

But now you speak up.

Janice:

(grins) Yes. I'm making up for it, for sure!

Aurora:

You're making up for it. Good!

Let's follow your story. What happened after the gunshot?

Justene:

I think that after that, people who were thinking of trying to escape dropped that idea.

WHAT HAPPENED AFTER THE GUNSHOT?

Aurora:

I can understand that.

When were you released?

Justene:

It was right before Chinese New Year, so January, February. I remember being released with my family, my mom, and the three kids.

My uncle wasn't released. They kept the men longer.

Aurora:

So you were released right before Chinese New Year.

Justene:

Yes. I remember I had just one set of clothes left by then. They took everything.

When I arrived in the concentration camp, I had two sets of clothes. I remember being able to take a shower and change my clothes. But by the time I left the concentration camp, I only had the clothes I was wearing.

In Vietnam at that time, you had to have your clothes made. You couldn't just go to a store and pick up a set of clothes off the rack.

So I remember after a couple of days, and I got a second set of clothes as my New Year's present that year. That was special.

Aurora:

When you were released from the concentration camp, did you feel euphoria, or were you just exhausted?

Justene:

We were happy to be released.

But my uncle was not released, so we were worried about him.

Aurora:

Where did you go?

Justene:

We returned to my grandparent's house.

Aurora:

What happened to your uncle?

Justene:

He got released a few months later.

So that was the first time I tried to escape.

Aurora:

What happened the next time you tried to escape?

WHAT HAPPENED THE NEXT TIME YOU TRIED TO ESCAPE?

Justene:

So after that first attempted escape, I went to back to school. Things were kind of normal.

About two years later, so 1985 or 1986, my mom got enough money again. I think my parents had an ice cream shop at the time. My mom saved up some money so that I could escape again, the second time.

Janice:

This time it was just Justene.

Justene:

There was some urgency because I was approaching the age where I was going to be enlisted.

My parents were really worried about what would happen to me if I was forced to join the army. They saved enough money to help me escape. But this time, there was only enough money for one person, so I would be escaping alone.

Aurora:

How old were you?

Justene:

I was 12, so it was four years later.

Aurora:

You're very bright. I'm guessing you weren't getting enough challenge at school, at the age of 12?

Justene:

I don't know what happened when I was younger. I wasn't a very bright student, to be completely honest.

Janice:
It's true.

Aurora:
(surprised) Maybe a lack of nutrition? That'll do it.

Janice:
I remember she got a lot of tutoring.

Justene:
My uncle, who was my math teacher, was upset with me most of the time.

Janice:
Yes.

Aurora:
Well, that's surprising. I would never have guessed. Okay, so you were not the best student as a kid?

Justene:
No, not as a kid. In the eighth grade, it just switched for me.

Aurora:
Eighth grade?

Justene:

Yes.

Aurora:

Well, I'm curious what shifted for you in eighth grade. But let's not jump ahead there yet.

Janice:

Let's go back.

Aurora:

Right. So your parents raised the money, thanks, perhaps, to the aunt in France and some ice cream shop profits?

Justene:

Yes.

Aurora:

They have just enough money for one escape, so your little sister Janice gets left behind. But they decide to try again.

Justene:

Yes, they pay for me to escape again.

Aurora:

What happened?

Justene:

This time, I escaped with my youngest aunt, my mom's youngest sister. It was just the two of us. We traveled for a long time. By bus, on foot, on bicycles, to a small town near a beach.

We've traveled by foot for two or three hours to get to this town. My aunt and I are hiding, waiting for nightfall, waiting for it to be dark.

When it was completely dark, around 10 pm, we crept onto the beach. But we never made it to the boat. Something happened.

Maybe the guard was watching us the entire time. We didn't have a window to escape.

Aurora:

You didn't have a chance.

Justene:

We didn't have a chance to escape in the dark. When the sun rose, my aunt and I and the rest of the people had to travel back another two, three hours by foot, and then we all got back on the bus.

I remember the sun was coming up, and it was a beautiful sunrise.

Aurora:
Interesting that you remember the sunrise.

Justene:
We didn't make it even to the boat this time.

Aurora:
But the money was spent?

Justene:
The money was spent.

Aurora:
Was a boat waiting there for you?

Justene:
I'm not sure. It was pitch dark, and I didn't see a boat. But we didn't have to pay for everything up front. There was an initial payment to get a spot on the boat, and then if we got through, the rest of the money had to be paid.

Aurora:
In these situations, you can't be sure if they will deliver what they promise.

Justene:
Right.

Aurora:

So, it was a beautiful sunrise. How did you feel? Were you happy about the sunrise? Or crushed because you didn't escape?

Justene:

Well, at 12, I understood my environment more clearly. There was not a whole lot of opportunity for me. My dad's background in the army definitely held me back. So I really wanted to escape.

I saw the money that my aunt was sending us from France, and I wanted to be like her. I wanted to escape so that I could help my family back home.

Aurora:

Right.

Justene:

So I was a bit disappointed.

Aurora:

That's an understatement: "a bit disappointed"! Then what happened?

Justene:

I traveled back to my grandparents. I knew that we were out of money, even though no one spoke about it.

I realized that I wouldn't have another chance to escape. Not then, maybe not ever.

> I REALIZED THAT I WOULDN'T HAVE ANOTHER CHANCE TO ESCAPE. NOT THEN, MAYBE NOT EVER

Justene:

Maybe that's why I focused more on school in grade 8. Before then, I wasn't a good student. I was distracted. But I knew that I didn't have any more money to escape. I started doing better in school.

Aurora:

It sounds like you made a decision.

I'm guessing here, you'll correct me if I'm wrong. Perhaps before the second failed attempt to escape, you were more of a child, having fun or being easily distracted.

Afterward, you realized the consequences. Your family was out of money, your opportunities were limited, you might never escape.

You faced reality, and you shifted to an adult perspective. "What do I need to do to survive and have more opportunities?" Then you changed your attitude about studying.

Justene:

Yes, I think so. I became a good student.

Aurora:

How did you feel when she came back, Janice? Were you upset that your bossy older sister was back? Or sad that she didn't escape?

Janice:

Actually, I didn't know that she was escaping. No one told us. No one in the neighborhood, not even our family.

Justene:

Whenever we planned to escape, it had to be kept top secret. It was very clandestine.

Aurora:

You wouldn't want anything to slip out.

Janice:

Right.

Justene:

After that, my aunt got to escape again. This time, she got through. I didn't even know about it. Every time we planned an escape, it was kept quiet.

Aurora:

Top secret.

Janice:

While my aunt was gone for a few days, I thought she went to visit our parents. I didn't know she was escaping.

Aurora:

That makes sense. The stakes are so high. You need to keep it hush-hush. Although that may have contributed to you feeling left out in the decision-making process once again.

Janice:

Yes. Exactly.

Aurora:

What happened next?

Justene:

I became a really good student. I excelled from that point on. In

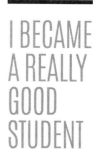

I BECAME A REALLY GOOD STUDENT

Vietnam, I got into AP classes in 10th and 11th grade.

Aurora:

You start taking the advanced placement (AP) classes.

Justene:

In just a short time, I turned into a really good student. I left Vietnam in 11th grade, so I was a junior in high school.

Somehow my mom found out that the US and Vietnam had an immigration program that allowed soldiers in the old army to immigrate to the US. The women in my family are strong.

Aurora:

With strong family values.

Justene:

From my grandmother, to my aunt, to my mother, all strong women.

My mom did all the paperwork. I don't know where she got the money, but we had to pay to apply, and she had to pay some more money for us to go. We were able to borrow money from a US charity, the Catholic Church, to buy our plane ticket.

Aurora:

So up until that point, it had been a real black mark against you that your father had been in the South Vietnamese army.

Then, the disadvantage turns into an advantage. It opens the door for you to immigrate to the US.

Janice:

Right.

Aurora:

And your mom was smart enough to notice and grab the opportunity.

Justene:

Yes. Four of us kids, and then my parents, so six of us get to go live in the US.

Aurora:

All together?

Janice:

By plane, all together.

Aurora:

Plane definitely is the way to go.

Janice:

But we still went to a concentration camp first.

Aurora:

What?!

Janice:

We were in a concentration camp in Thailand for about two months.

Aurora:

You stayed in Thailand for two months before going to the US?

Justene:

We went from Vietnam to Thailand, and we had to stay there for two months for some reason. I think the paperwork wasn't complete, or there was some technical issue that we weren't able to go to the US right away.

Aurora:

And that was like a concentration camp in your view?

Janice:
It was a concentration camp!

Justene:
You're not allowed to go outside.

Janice:
You're surrounded by a fence.

Justene:
Gate and guard.

Janice:
Guards with guns.

Aurora:
That sounds terrifying.

Janice:
Yes, I was only ten years old. I didn't even really know what it meant to leave Vietnam. I just knew, the last few days in Vietnam, my parents were trying to pack, and trying to get money, and trying to get passport photos. They were doing a lot of things out of the ordinary.

But they still didn't tell me that we're leaving the country. No one told me anything!

Aurora:

I notice a bit of resentment about that.

Janice:

It's important to me to know what's going on.

Aurora:

That's why you tell people what's going on, today, as a dentist.

Janice:

Yes. I want my patients to understand what's going on, and feel respected.

Aurora:

That makes sense. Okay, so back to Thailand, to the concentration camp. What happened?

Janice:

We got there late. It was night time, and my brothers and I, we're goofing around, we're playing, the three of us. I was ten, he was nine, and then the other one's seven. So we were just kids, and we are playing around, goofing off. I remember my sister getting upset with us, because we're not listening to her.

Aurora:
You were 16, Justene?

Justene:
Yes.

Aurora:
There's a big difference between 10 and 16.

Janice:
Right.

So then we got in, and they gave us a station with a bed, and we have to share among the six of us. My parents told me we were supposed to be there for a week or so, just to get the paperwork done before we continue our adventure.

But one week turned into two weeks, three weeks, four weeks.

My parents kept checking in, but they didn't release us. We were stuck there. They just gave us rice and eggs. So that's what you have breakfast, lunch, and dinner.

After the first week, I thought, "Oh my God, I can't take the smell anymore." It was horrific.

Aurora:

When we were in Indonesia, it was Nasi Goreng, breakfast, lunch, and dinner. It's stir-fried rice and whatever else is handy. Usually eggs and some vegetables, perhaps a bit of meat, and peanut sauce.

I can see why you'd get weary of just rice and eggs pretty quickly.

Janice:

They had other food, but you had to pay for it. Sometimes, maybe once a week, my mom would buy some food, so that we would get some other protein.

Aurora:

What a story! Speaking of food, have a snack. How about some nuts?

(passing snacks around)

I want to hear the rest of your story and don't want you fading. You must have been malnourished as a kid.

Janice:

Yes. I was.

Aurora:

How did you deal with food?

Janice:

Ever since I was young, I remember sharing food with my little brother. At the concentration camp, either he would eat, or I
would eat. We would have to take turns.

If my baby brother doesn't eat, he gets
fussy and starts crying. So a lot of time I had
to wait patiently for him to finish before I
could eat. Even though I'm starving.

Aurora:

You were patient and generous, even as
a child.

Janice:

When we were growing up, my younger
brother James was always hungry. He's a boy,
he's growing. A lot of times, he finished his
food and he would look around, still hungry.
I would eat just enough, and then I would
give him my food. Then my third brother,
my youngest brother, came along, and I had
to share with him, too!

Aurora:

What was your typical food in Vietnam with your grandparents?

Janice:

We had breakfast, lunch, dinner. My grandma would usually cook lunch and dinner for us. Rice, different side dishes, and fruit. I liked the food she made, but I don't like rice. But rice is what is going to keep me full, so I tried to eat it.

I DON'T LIKE RICE

I was always watching to make sure my brothers were okay. If they still seemed hungry after they ate their food, I would share my food with them.

Aurora:

So you had a caring, nurturing energy. Like a mother.

Janice:

Yes, because neither my mother nor my father were with us. They lived in a small town in Vietnam.

Justene:

I was six when Janice was born. After nine months or so, Janice got to come and live with my grandparents and me in Saigon. Our parents stayed in the small town of Nha Trang. And then a year later James was born. After nine months, James got to join my grandparents, Janice and me in Saigon. Our mom and dad stayed in Nha Trang.

Then two years later, my youngest brother was born and my grandmother says, "That's it. He cannot come."

Aurora:

Your grandparents drew the line at three kids. I don't blame them!

Janice:

Right. The fourth one did not get to come.

Justene:

Our grandmother had her hands full taking care of three of us. So, Janice, James and I are a lot closer because we grew up together. Every once in a while our parents would visit us.

Janice:

Maybe twice a year we would see our baby brother John and our parents.

Justene:

My grandma taught me how to write the alphabet when I was 2 or 3 years old. She would hold my hands and help me write the alphabet.

When Janice was about 2 or 3 years old, I taught her how to write. I was eight. My grandma helped me show my little sister how to write the alphabet.

Aurora:

We learn best when we teach. Your grand–mother is wise.

Justene:

Yes, she is. Then, after teaching Janice, I taught James.

Our youngest brother John didn't get to come to Saigon, so I didn't teach him. I saw him only a couple of times a year. When we left Vietnam in 1991, John was seven years old.

Aurora:

Your grandparents raised you—they must be like parents to you.

Justene:

I have a really good family. We all have good family values. No one in my family ever got divorced, and as Janice said, we always share things with each other.

Aurora:

Even when it's a matter of keeping body and soul together, you share. Food was scarce.

Janice:

It was.

Aurora:

Well, tell me about malnutrition. I'm not a nutrition expert, but in times past when sailors would sail across the ocean, they didn't understand about the need for vitamin C, and so the sailors would get scurvy, and their teeth would fall out. No vitamin C, no teeth!

Janice:

True.

Aurora:

Or people would get Ricketts and crooked legs from malnutrition. So what happened to your health and teeth from having to survive primarily on rice?

Justene:

We didn't have a lot, but my grandmother tried to make it bearable.

We did have a lot of rice, which is just carbs. Not a whole lot of vegetables or proteins. Meat was expensive. Even fish was expensive. But my grandmother managed to get us a bit of extra food.

Aurora:

Your grandmother was an educated woman. She was a teacher, so she was probably aware of the need for vegetables and protein?

Justene:

Yes. She was the reason that we felt more fortunate than other kids in our neighborhood.

Janice:

When I was younger, I was very skinny. Compared to all the other kids in the neighborhood I was very small for my age.

Aurora:

Probably due to lack of nutrition?

Janice:

Yes.

Aurora:

So you're in the concentration camp in Thailand, waiting to go to the United States.

Tell me about arriving in the United States. Where did you arrive? How did it feel to go on a plane? How did your lives change?

Stranger in a Strange Land: USA

Justene:
I had had some English classes, for maybe a year. My mom was preparing us.

Aurora:
Your mom had foresight.

Justene:
Yeah, she was smart. So I understood a little bit of English. I remember on the flight, we were trying to figure it out.

We knew "chicken" and "fish". My mom was always concerned that we get enough food. When they offered food, we would always take it. And that came from not having enough. If we didn't finish it, she would keep it for us to eat later. So I remember that part of being on the airplane.

Justene:
One funny story about arriving in America—we landed first in Portland Ore-

gon International airport en route to San Francisco.

My brother saw an apple for the very first time. He would not leave. My youngest brother just stood there and stared at the apple.

Aurora:
He was mesmerized.

Justene:
Airport food is expensive. But my brother was entranced by the apple. So then my mom had to buy him an apple at the airport kiosk. And he was really, really happy just having that red apple.

Aurora:
It's amazing how much we take for granted. Today in the US, we can have almost any fruit or vegetable, any day of the year. No matter what the season.

But it wasn't always that way. I remember my mother, who was born in 1933, telling me how excited she was to get an orange in her Christmas stocking. That was a big deal at Christmas time—each of her brothers and sisters got one orange. One Mandarin orange—that was very special.

Janice:
Oh.

Aurora:
These days, we take so many things for granted.

Justene:
Sometimes we cherish little things, that emotionally or spiritually that have a big impact. Like the time that I get to spend with my family now. I cherish that.

Aurora:
That is precious.

So, arriving in America, you don't speak English except for "fish" and "chicken"?

Justene:
True.

Aurora:
And you've never seen an apple before. So you're in for quite the shock, I imagine, in San Francisco?

Janice:
We got there, and it was very cold. Vietnam temperature is above 90 degrees at all times.

Justene:
San Francisco, June 1991, it was cold.

Aurora:
Cold and windy.

Justene:
So that was my first experience with America. You know, we hear things about America, and this is like freedom, not Communist, and we looked forward to being in the US.

We arrived in San Francisco, and I thought, "Oh my God, we're going to die." I thought I would freeze to death.

Aurora:
Brrrrr. Where did you go?

Justene:
My grandmother's sister worked for the Bank of America, so she sponsored us. So we stayed with her for a few months before we moved out to Los Angeles with my uncle.

Aurora:

How old were you when you arrived in Los Angeles?

Justene:

I was 16. I was a junior in high school, and Janice was 10.

Aurora:

Los Angeles is different from San Francisco in some major ways. What was your experience?

Janice:

Everything was different for me. My experience coming over here was slightly different from Justene's. I didn't know where I was going. I didn't know about America. I had no clue what was going on. I just followed my parents and my sister.

For example, I'd never been on an airplane before. The air in the airplane made me feel dizzy. I didn't like the smell of the air itself. It was making me feel sick.

Aurora:

That airplane air can be nauseating.

Janice:
Yes. I didn't like being on the airplane seat because it was closer to the air vent, so I liked being underneath the chair. And I would hide under there.

Aurora:
You were tiny!

Janice:
Yes, I could fit anywhere.

Aurora:
You could sleep under the chair.
(laughs)

You don't see many people making that choice in an airplane.

Justene:
(smiles)
We were the only ones, I think.

Janice:
I'm sure the other people on the airplane were looking at me. I didn't care, I was just going to make myself comfortable. So I was underneath my parent's feet under the chair in the airplane.

Once we got to the airport, I remember my brother being amazed by the apple. I was amazed by all the people.

I'd never seen any other ethnicity. My whole world up until that point was filled with people who looked just like me.

Americans towered over me, like giants. I thought, "holy moly, where am I?"

> AMERICANS TOWERED OVER ME LIKE GIANTS. I THOUGHT, "HOLY MOLY, WHERE AM I?"

Aurora:

It's as though your whole life was vanilla ice cream and then you realize there are dozens of flavors of ice cream.

Janice:

Exactly.

Then we went to see our grandma and aunt and uncle in San Francisco. I was freezing. I was so skinny I felt the cold right to the bone. It was painfully cold.

Aurora:

It was a shock to your system to go from 90-degree weather to 55-degree weather.

Janice:

Yes, exactly. I didn't want to go outside, I just wanted to stay inside.

Aurora:

Didn't they give you warmer clothes?

Janice:

No, they didn't.

Justene:

We eventually got some.

Janice:

Eventually, my mom gave me more clothes. We didn't pack warm clothes because we didn't have cold weather in Vietnam.

Aurora:

Right. A different climate.

Janice:

Yeah. We didn't go shopping. People donated clothes.

Justene:

My mom would go to church, and then they'd donate clothes for us to wear. But the first few days, we didn't have warm clothing. We only had sandals and shorts and thin cotton shirts, and it was freezing.

Aurora:

What's your next memory from arriving in the United States?

Janice:

Getting into a car. I'd never been in a car. Back in Vietnam, we have bicycles or motor-cycles. So you're always outdoors. So being inside this little box was new, I didn't know what a car was.

Aurora:

Were you excited about the adventure, or frightened?

Janice:

I was curious. What does a car do? I didn't know it would take you places. I had never been in a car.

IT WAS LIKE A "STRANGER IN A STRANGE LAND" ADVENTURE

Aurora:

It was like a "Stranger in a Strange Land" adventure—as if you had arrived on another planet?

Janice:

Yes, I felt like that. Once I got inside the car, I didn't like the air.

Aurora:

You're sensitive to the way things smell.

Janice:

Yeah, the smell made me feel sick. Even though I was cold, I had to put down the window. I'd rather have the cold air than the stale air inside the car.

Aurora:

On another note, maybe that's one of the reasons why, when you gave me the tour of your offices at A+ Family Dentistry yesterday, you showed me the water purifiers.

Maybe your sensitivity to smell—and also your childhood experience of not being told what was happening—now makes you determined to reassure your patients and make sure everything is transparent.

I've never seen that before, where a dentist shows patients how purified the water is, and the special water filtration system you had installed. I appreciated that.

What about you, Justene? What stood out to you when you arrived in the States?

Justene:

It was an accumulation of a many different things, but I adapted quickly.

The food was different. In Vietnam, we never had tomato sauce. My aunt and uncle, they ordered pizza and told us, "This is really good!" But we couldn't eat it. I would just eat the crust on the outside of a pizza.

Janice:

Or burgers. We could only eat French fries, we couldn't eat hamburgers.

Justene:

Yeah. I remember I would tell my mom, "I just want rice. Can you give me rice?"

Aurora:

But you don't like rice!

Justene:

Exactly. But it was familiar.

Then everything changed when school started. I got used to school very, very quickly.

Aurora:

Hold everything, how'd you get used to it "very, very quickly" when you didn't speak English?

Justene:

I spoke it a little bit. I was good at math, so I was in an AP Calculus class when I first started in high school in the US. My math teacher was kind. He took me under his wing and made sure everything was okay for me.

What stood out to me was the student attitude here in America. In classrooms, students would talk while the teacher was talking. The students would have their feet on the table. That is not acceptable in Vietnam at all! So that disrespect was weird for me.

In Vietnam, we respect all teachers. I don't like the disrespectful attitude towards teachers here in America.

I took the AP Calculus class, and I took a lot of English. I had three English classes at the same time.

Aurora:
English as a second language, or English classes? Which?

Justene:
Both. I took English as a second language and regular English and AP English all at the same time.

Aurora:
You took AP English? Wow.

Justene:
I didn't need to study anything else. I was able to transfer my credits from Vietnam. I had already taken geometry, calculus, physics, chemistry. So I took three English classes at the same time through my junior and senior year. A lot of English classes!

Aurora:
Well, that's what you needed. But still, it must have been challenging. Or did you thrive?

Justene:
No, it was challenging. I had some Viet-namese friends in high school. There was a group of six of us. I didn't have American friends in high school. I remember we were laughed at sometimes.

Aurora:
Ow.

Justene:
But at the time the American kids were making fun of me, I didn't understand it, so it was okay.

Aurora:
Were you speaking English or Vietnamese with your Vietnamese friends in high school?

Justene:
A little bit of both. We were all trying to learn English. Some had been here longer, so they spoke more English. So we were trying. I was trying.

Aurora:
In high school, I felt like a misfit at times. Often, I was the smartest—or at least the

most outspoken—kid in the class, and that didn't make me popular with the other kids.

I had a different background. I had traveled more, had a different life experience. I loved learning. I still do.

But how about you? Did you feel like you didn't belong? Did you feel lonely? Or like a "stranger in a strange land" in high school? Or did you feel, "I'm good, I understand calculus, I'm taking English, I have some friends."

Justene:

I wasn't so worried about it socially at that point. There was so much for me to learn.

Moving to America was such an enormous change from Vietnam. I was trying to understand my new surroundings. I was busy studying.

My mom was working at home at the time as well, and she needed my help. Being a teenager, I didn't particularly want to help my mom, but I had to, you know? So I helped. We sewed a lot of clothes at home to make ends meet.

I was busy with school, learning English, helping my mom, helping Janice and my brothers, and learning how to drive.

Aurora:
Learning how to drive? Your aunt and uncle had a car?

Justene:
My uncle had a truck.

My parents, again I don't know how they did it, my mom worked full time, and then some. My dad went to school to be an electrician.

Aurora:
Good for him.

Justene:
So my mom supported the whole family. My dad learned how to drive first. Somehow they saved up enough money to buy a used car for me when I turned 18. My dad was going to school and driving the kids. I don't know how my Mom did it.

Aurora:

I admire your parents' priorities, grit and determination.

Justene:

Me, too.

Aurora:

You mentioned that they don't speak English very well even today, right?

Justene:

Even today they don't.

Aurora:

So they were much more isolated than you.

Justene:

Absolutely. My dad made the decision not to live in an area saturated with Vietnamese because he loved us and wanted us to learn English. So we lived in an area with few Vietnamese people. It made it more difficult for my parents.

Aurora:

More difficult for them, much easier for you. Once again, they were thinking about you.

Justene:

Absolutely.

Aurora:

I admire that.

Justene:

Same here.

Aurora:

Today, in 2017, most people are thinking about themselves. They're thinking about the next day, or the next month, the short term.

Your parents took the long view of life. They were anticipating the future. When you were 10 years old, they were worried about what would happen when you were 18. They didn't want you to be drafted into the Vietnamese army.

They were saving up. They were thinking not only about next year, but the next decade, and the decade after that.

They were thinking about what's best for you, and repeatedly choosing more challenge, more adversity for themselves, to give you and your siblings a better future.

Justene:

Absolutely. Absolutely.

Let's go back a bit. I want to share that we were on food stamps when we got here. And even then, I didn't want to be on food stamps. Do you remember that, Janice?

I DIDN'T WANT TO BE ON FOOD STAMPS

Janice:

I remember we were on food stamps, but I didn't know what that meant. I just knew that when I went to the supermarket to help my mom, and I would have to go and match the picture. I didn't know how to read English yet, so I would just look at the picture and match it and get it for my mom.

Aurora:

Food stamps would buy basics like bread, milk, eggs, and things like that, right?

Justene:

Right. For like the first few months it didn't bother me, and then I started getting used to seeing other people pay with money. I remember a conversation about all the Vietnamese staying at home or getting paid under the table and not ever getting off of food stamps after being here for 20 years!

That's not the way that I think. That's not how my dad thinks. My dad took a couple of years to study and become an electrician. It was a more difficult choice. He sacrificed earning money right away to go to school. He was able to get a better job later, as an electrician. After a couple of years, he was a very good electrician, and he worked with a company.

Aurora:
Again it was short term pain for long-term gain. He was consistent.

Justene:
Yeah, that's big in my family. Talking to you now, I realize that we operate that way, too. We prioritize the long term.

Aurora:
It's a default setting in your family. Yeah. In fact, it relates to dentistry, because it is short-term pain for long-term gain.

Justene:

Not much pain. We numb the patients, so they experience very little pain.

Aurora:

Not much pain, but the inconvenience of taking an hour or two off work to take care of your teeth. But then it can change your life in the long term. You can get 10, 20, 30 years more health and vitality by taking care of your mouth. You can reverse the signs of aging with a beautiful smile, and that makes you look younger and feel younger, for a long time.

So this focus on the long-term relates to your family, and also to your career as a dentist. That's interesting.

So your father chose to study, short-term pain, but then he had a higher income, long-term gain.

Justene:

Exactly. I think it took me six months to a year to get used to going to the supermarket and seeing all the people paying with money and we were paying with food stamps. I didn't like it. That's not going to be our future.

Aurora:

It sounds like you make a decision. What changed after that?

Justene:

I helped my mom out more. She wasn't happy with the sewing that she was doing at the time because it was a lot of work for little pay. But she was doing it for the family. So I helped her more. And within two years we got off of food stamps completely.

Aurora:

She was supporting the family because your father was studying, so not earning money.

Justene:

Yes, for the first two years.

Aurora:

And were you still living with your aunt and uncle?

Justene:

We had our own place. My uncle found us a three-bedroom house in Los Angeles, and there was a room that mom worked in.

Aurora:

Thank you for sharing your fascinating story.

I'm noticing turning points in your story. Something happens—or you see things differently—and then you shift. For example, the second time you were caught attempting to escape from Vietnam, you shifted and became a more serious and diligent student.

When you arrived in the US, you didn't know the meaning of food stamps at first. But then you observed other people were paying with money. And you also noticed that some people had been here for twenty years and were still paying with food stamps. You decided that you didn't want to be on food stamps like them. Then you made a choice. You shifted and worked harder to help your mom. You did well in high school.

What happened next? You went to a university because you're a dentist today. You're both dentists. How did that happen?

Grit & Dental School

Justene:

Right after high school, I didn't have money for college.

In Vietnam, either you know somebody, and not having a mark against your family, and you get in. But I had a mark against me because my Dad was in the Vietnamese army, so college would not have been in my future if I was still in Vietnam.

But in the US, I had the opportunity to go to college. And I was determined to go. But I didn't have any money.

So, when I graduated from high school, I signed up for the army.

I WAS DETERMINED TO GO TO COLLEGE. BUT I DIDN'T HAVE ANY MONEY. SO I SIGNED UP FOR THE ARMY

Aurora:

What?! After your parents came all the way to the United States to avoid you getting drafted into the army, you signed up for the Army?

Justene:
My parents were not happy about it.

Aurora:
I guess not. Why did you do that?

Justene:
Because I didn't know any other way to get the money I needed for college.

Aurora:
So again, short-term pain, long-term gain.

Justene:
I didn't understand government support, or state grants, or loans at the time. And my parent barely spoke English, so I didn't have a whole lot of guidance.

Aurora:
It wasn't normal to get student loans in Vietnam?

Justene:
Right. So I graduated from high school. In June, I turned 18. I learned that I could make my own decisions when I was 18 years old.

So I signed up for the Army so that I could go to college.

Aurora:
Your parents must have been upset.

Justene:
Yes. You can imagine that conversation. They weren't happy.

Aurora:
I guess not! We escaped from Vietnam to save you from the army—and now you're going into the American Army?!

Justene:
We argued. But I was determined to go to college, and it was the only way. So, I applied for colleges. I applied to UC Berkeley. I got rejected. I applied to several schools. I got rejected. Finally, I got accepted at San Francisco State University.

Aurora:

You were freezing the last time you were in San Francisco.

Justene:

That was the only school that accepted me. So it was a way to achieve my dream of going to university, even if it is cold and windy. Also, San Francisco State was near my grandma in Oakland.

Once I got accepted, I did the paperwork, and I get to financial aid and step by step, I figured out that I could borrow money for school. So then I didn't want to go into the Army anymore.

Aurora:

What happened?

Justene:

I worked with some counselors and they helped me get out of the contract with the Army. That was a relief. I hadn't gone through boot camp or anything yet, the army hadn't paid for anything for school. So I got out of the Army and went to San Francisco State for four years.

Aurora:
What did you study?

Justene:
Biochemistry.

Aurora:
Biochemistry—you didn't choose some-thing easy.

Justene:
I'm still learning a lot of English, and get-ting used to the culture and being on my own in the dorms. So I was busy with that. In my second year of college, I volunteered at the hospital at UC San Francisco, UCSF. They have a hospital and a medical-dental school. I wanted to get into health care at the time.

Aurora:
At the time you were thinking to become a doctor?

Justene:
Yes, so I volunteered on the UCSF cancer floor.

Aurora:

I've been on those cancer floors. It can be heart-wrenching. My mother died of cancer.

Justene:

I had the idea of becoming a medical doctor. But volunteering at the hospital there, it was a bit sad even though doctors do heroic things and save patients. But it didn't really fit with my energy level. You know?

Aurora:

I do.

Justene:

By this point, I had learned more English. I liked having more American friends and I getting used to this culture. It was becoming more comfortable living here. I was coming out of my shell a lot more, being away from my parents, with the freedom to do things on my own.

Aurora:

Were you a wild girl at this point, or you were still "Miss Studious"?

Justene:

No, I was still really studious.

Aurora:

Did you consider other disciplines in medicine? Like pediatrics or something else?

Justene:

At that time, I worked for a couple of dentists—a husband and wife. I got to see how dentistry is still in health care. But it's a lot lighter, and patients come back more regularly instead of just one time.

Aurora:

You can develop relationships with your patients.

Justene:

I really like to get to know people, and have relationships over many years. So I worked at the dentistry office and I really, really liked it.

Aurora:

Was it hard to get into dentistry school?

I LIKE TO GET TO KNOW PEOPLE, AND HAVE RELATIONSHIPS OVER MANY YEARS. SO I WORKED AT THE DENTISTRY OFFICE AND I REALLY, REALLY LIKED IT

Justene:

It was competitive, but I had good grades in college. So getting in wasn't too difficult for me.

Aurora:

Where did you study?

Justene:

The University of Southern California, it's a great dental school.

Aurora:

You realized that you wanted to be a dentist, not a doctor.

Justene:

Yes, when I was working for a dentist I enjoyed dealing with people. I liked having ongoing relationships with patients.

Aurora:

You graduated from USC after studying for four years. Did it take you a long time to open your own dentistry practice?

Justene:

No, that's when my entrepreneurial spirit came in. I graduated August 2002. I was waiting for my license while I was opening my office at the same time.

Aurora:

That was quick. You're an entrepreneur.

Justene:

I didn't know any better at the time.

Aurora:

That's how most entrepreneurs start. They have no idea what they're getting into.

Justene:

True! My husband graduated a year ahead of me, so he had been a dentist for one year. (We were boyfriend and girlfriend at the time, we were engaged to get married.)

He had been practicing for a little bit less than one year when I graduated. I was waiting for my license and building my first practice at the same time.

Aurora:

Like anybody in a new business, I'm sure you made a lot of rookie mistakes?

Justene:

Absolutely.

Aurora:

Now that you have learned from them, you can teach other dentists how to avoid those expensive mistakes.

Justene:

Yes, at some point soon, we want to help other dentists build thriving practices. So they don't have empty chairs—like we had at the beginning. It took us a while to learn how to run a successful seven-figure business.

Aurora:

I'm just guessing here, but so many dentists who open a clinic have just learned about being a dentist, but they don't know how to run a business. Probably a lot of them go bankrupt?

Justene:

Absolutely. All that equipment is expensive.

> WE WANT TO HELP OTHER DENTISTS BUILD THRIVING 7-FIGURE PRACTICES. SO THEY DON'T HAVE EMPTY CHAIRS— LIKE WE HAD AT THE BEGINNING

Janice:

I think the majority of dentists don't reach their full potential. In my experience, the general public is not getting the service that they should get, because of dentists' inability to communicate.

Aurora:

It's easy for somebody who is skilled as a dentist, doctor, or another kind of expert to lack communication skills. A successful entrepreneur needs additional skills: communication, marketing, management, finance, sales.

Janice:

Absolutely.

Aurora:

So many people have a negative opinion of sales. Done with integrity, selling is serving. When a dentist—or anyone—is offering the right solution it's not manipulation; it's serving. You're giving them information that they need. You're letting them know the short-term and long-term health consequences if they don't take care of their teeth now. They may not have any teeth later. They might have to get dentures.

Grandma, Can I Have Your Teeth?

Justene:

My grandmother had dentures. I was four or five years old, that was before Janice came along. This is my first memory about teeth.

Every morning, in the kitchen, I would watch my grandma take her teeth out. I would watch her every single move, because my parents weren't around, just my grandmother. And I would watch her every single morning taking her teeth out, brushing them outside, putting them back in.

Aurora:

What did you think about that?

Justene:

I assumed that everyone would lose their teeth when they get older. You know? My grandma was probably in her late 50s at this time.

I would ask my grandma, "Grandma, when you pass away can I have your teeth?"

AS A CHILD I WAS FASCINATED WITH MY GRANDMA'S DENTURES. I ASKED HER, "GRANDMA, WHEN YOU PASS AWAY CAN I HAVE YOUR TEETH?"

Aurora:
You were practical.

Justene:
Yes. I watched those dentures like a hawk. I wanted to make sure that I inherited that set of teeth. So that was my first memory of teeth.

Aurora:
How did she respond, do you remember?

Justene:
She said, "Sure," or something like that. But I was very determined watching that set of teeth.

Aurora:
It sounds like your interest in teeth started in that kitchen with your grandmother and her dentures. I can imagine a four-year-old being fascinated, "Oh, these things come out? Who knew?"

What about you, Janice? What's your first memory with teeth?

Janice:

When I was six or seven years old, my baby teeth were coming in. This was in Vietnam, and we didn't have the money to go to the dentist. My grandpa (who was not a dentist) would try to pull out my baby teeth because my adult teeth were trying to come out, but there was no room for them.

I remember my mom was visiting us, and she took my brother somewhere. I wanted to go with them, but she left me alone with my grandpa.

My grandpa put me on a chair and he held me tight. I didn't know what was going on, so I started crying. Then he pulled a tool, like big pliers. Then he pulled my baby teeth out!

Aurora:

Ow.

Janice:

It was painful.

Aurora:

Yes. You must have been frightened.

Janice:

Yes, I was, because I didn't know what was going on. What was he doing and why? He took control, and he pulled my baby teeth out. I was screaming at the top of my lungs trying to get away, and I couldn't.

Aurora:

How old were you then?

Janice:

Around three or four.

Aurora:

That experience probably contributes to you being so kind and gentle now that you are a dentist. You take the time to explain things to your patients.

Janice:

Yes, I always want my patients to know what is happening and why. I don't do dentistry by surprise.

I remember when I came over to America, I didn't know how to brush my teeth. I don't think I ever owned a toothbrush. And the whole time during concentration camp, I don't think I ever brushed my teeth.

Justene:
I remember grandma taught me how to brush my teeth.

Janice:
But I was not responsible.

Aurora:
You have beautiful teeth now, but you did not have beautiful teeth earlier?

Janice:
No, I didn't. I had a lot of dental work when I came to America. I had many cavities. My mouth would hurt when I ate certain food.

When I got here to America, I went to the dentist, and I didn't know what was going on. I would get drilling, lots of metal fillings. Some were more painful than others.

Aurora:
So you had some early traumatic experiences with dentistry—making you committed to helping others in a gentle and communicative way today.

Janice:

Exactly. I had lots of cavities. I didn't know how to brush my teeth. I had a lot of plaque even when I went to college.

I admired people who had nice teeth. I wondered what they were doing differently, and what I could do to have a nicer smile.

> I ADMIRED PEOPLE WHO HAD NICE TEETH. I WONDERED WHAT THEY WERE DOING DIFFERENTLY, AND WHAT I COULD DO TO HAVE A NICER SMILE

Aurora:

How did you get your teeth so beautiful now?

Janice:

After lots of care!

When Justene became a dentist, I started to learn more about dentistry. I would volunteer. In dental school, I learned how to brush and floss my teeth properly.

Justene:

But you had braces earlier, though.

Janice:

Yes, I had braces when I was in college, at the end of my first year. And with braces, I didn't know how to brush my teeth either. I didn't know how to care for them, or any of that.

Aurora:
Did you have the metal kind, that looks like a grill? They didn't have Invisalign® yet, right?

Janice:
They didn't have Invisalign® back then.

Aurora:
What prompted you to become a dentist, Janice? Was it that early experience with your teeth being yanked out, or was it following in your big sister's footsteps, or something else?

WHAT PROMPTED YOU TO BECOME A DENTIST, JANICE?

Janice:
I've always wanted to help other people. I knew I wanted to do something in healthcare, and I volunteered.

I worked at an optometry office when I was in high school. I thought it was easy and fun, and I liked helping others. But after a while, I found that it was boring.

When I got to college, I thought that I wanted to become a doctor.

Aurora:

(grins)

That sounds familiar.

Janice:

I volunteered in a hospital. Not cancer care, like Justene. I volunteered in ER—in Emergency.

Aurora:

Emergency—that sounds more challenging than oncology.

Janice:

It was very challenging because there are so many trauma cases coming and going. So many people are suffering. I thought, "Oh my God, there's just so much to do."

Aurora:

Not a very pretty place to be, the ER. So how quickly did you realize, "Hmm. I don't know about this doctor thing. I think I might choose a new career path."

Janice:

It didn't take long for me to realize that the ER wasn't for me.

Then I tried pharmacy. It's just one after the other trying to see what fits.

Aurora:

You were resisting following in your sister's footsteps with the pharmacy move.

Janice:

Exactly.

Aurora:

I'd like to circle back. What tips do you have for people with braces?

WHAT TIPS DO YOU HAVE FOR PEOPLE WITH BRACES?

Janice:

I have a little story. When I was in college, I had my first set of braces, but I didn't wear my retainer. So my teeth started to shift back. They weren't straight anymore.

Janice:

So it wasn't until 2013—when I was a dentist already—that I started talking to other people about having straighter teeth. I looked in the mirror and saw that I didn't have straight teeth. I wanted to be a good role model for my patients. So I decided to put braces back on.

Aurora:

Wow, good for you! Because you didn't wear your retainer, you needed to get braces again.

Janice:

Yes. And I skipped that. So the point of my story is to tell people who have braces to wear their retainer!

Aurora:

Warning: wear your retainer.

If you skip one step, you don't get the desired result. If you're baking bread, but you skip the yeast, it doesn't go well. If you brush your teeth, but you skip flossing, it doesn't go well. If you think about going to the dentist, but you don't pick up the phone and call, it doesn't go well.

Janice:
Exactly.

Aurora:
When you were little, how did you brush your teeth?

Justene:
In Vietnam, we had toothbrushes. We didn't have toothbrushes in the concentration camp in Thailand. We rinsed with water.

Janice:
If we had any water.

Aurora:
What's interesting is that you two have had so many challenges. Different people have different challenges. It's the human experience.

But not many of your patients can say they were in a concentration camp, had malnutrition, and didn't have a toothbrush. In spite of all of these challenges, you both have beautiful teeth now because you learned some new things, and were proactive.

Justene:

Yes, we're lucky we took action before it was too late.

Aurora:

What are the keys to a healthy smile after the age of 40?

Keys to a Healthy Smile After 40

Justene:

Let's start with what to do in your 30s and 40s. Most people start having a family in their 30s. When you have a family, and you have children, it's still essential to take care of your own teeth.

Most parents don't think about it, so they care for the newborn and they neglect their own health or dental care. They don't realize that having poor oral health (like cavities or a gum infection) could be transferred to their babies.

Aurora:

That's shocking!

Justene:

Absolutely. We take ongoing education to keep up with the latest studies and science.

I think it was in the last 5 to 10 years that better saliva testing identified 13 kinds of bacteria that cause gum disease.

It makes sense, when you get a common cold, virus and bacteria transfer when you're in close proximity to another person. So gum disease and cavities are caused by specific bacteria.

Newborns get their first teeth at six months. I've seen new parents taking good care of their children but neglecting their own oral care. They're not aware that having cavities or a gum infection in their own mouth could cause problems for their baby.

Aurora:

And parents should be good role models. Children mimic their parents.

Janice:

Absolutely. I see that when parents come in, and they are scared of going to the dentist themselves, I advise them to be a bit more relaxed. Children will tune in to their parent's emotions. You don't want to teach your children that it is threatening to go to the dentist. They can sense if you are nervous.

Aurora:

Yesterday, I noticed that you put your patients at ease, you take your time, you show them around, and they get comfortable. I'm sure in your office, people are much more relaxed.

In general, what do you recommend if people are apprehensive?

Janice:

If the parent feels apprehensive when it comes to a dental appointment, I suggest they don't bring their child with them.

That way the child doesn't get the wrong message. And that way, the dentist can help the patient overcome their anxiety without the distraction of a fussy child. For your child's sake, you should overcome your fear.

What is causing your fear? For some, it is the unknown. For others, it's the needle, pain, or noise. The anticipation of pain is usually more painful than the actual experience. People fear different things. I ask my patients what's the root of their fear. Then I can help them.

Aurora:

In my experience, just thinking about something doesn't make the fear abate, but if you just do it, the fear releases. "Feel the fear and do it anyway" as Susan Jefferson says in her book by the same title. See the dentist and your fear will abate.

Janice:
I find that most of the time, people just fear the unknown. That's why we tell patients what we are going to do before we do it. The majority of the time, that's really helpful.

Other people are afraid of the shot. We have differ-ent ways of handling that fear. We use a topical cream to get the gum numb, and that makes the shot painless. Other people are afraid of the noise of the drill. In that case, our patients can listen to music with noise reduction headphones.

MOST OF THE TIME, PEOPLE JUST FEAR THE UNKNOWN. THAT'S WHY WE TELL PATIENTS WHAT WE ARE GOING TO DO BEFORE WE DO IT

Aurora:
You offer noise reduction headphones?

Janice:
Yes, and we play music.

Aurora:

That's smart.

Janice:

It sounds very different when you have noise reduction headphones.

Aurora:

Are there other dentists who provide noise reduction headphones and the music? Is that common? I've never heard of that before.

Janice:

Some dentists really care and take the time to go the extra mile. The patient can be in the chair for a couple of hours. We want them to be comfortable.

Aurora:

Hence, you provide massaging chairs. Awesome idea! I've never seen that in a dentist's office before either.

Justene:

When we give a shot, we do a little technique to distract the patient, so they don't focus on the shot. Instead, they focus on our massage.

Aurora:

You give them a little massage?

Justene:

Yes, on the shoulder. I hear a lot of good things about it. Patients say they didn't even feel the needle. Their attention was on the massage

Aurora:

What other suggestions do you have for people in their 30s?

Janice:

In your 30s, people are starting their careers. You might not realize it, but your smile matters a lot in job interviews. People who are embarrassed about their teeth tend not to smile very much, and can seem unfriendly.

You want to feel confident smiling. Nowadays, having really crooked or yellow teeth can affect your ability to get a job. Making a good first impression matters.

Aurora:

It's very important. And you're always interviewing for something. You're interviewing to get a job or get a promotion. You're interviewing for a date. You're interviewing for a scholarship.

Janice:
I think people in their 30s do not realize how much having a beautiful smile can improve their life.

Aurora:
A nice smile gives you more confidence, which also increases your probability of success.

Janice:
Absolutely. People pay attention to the way they dress, having the right clothing, the right hair, right nails, right makeup. But they don't realize that a healthy smile can enhance their look.

Aurora:
That's so true, we get our hair done, we get our nails done, we get a new outfit—but then we don't take care of our teeth.

Your teeth are an asset. In southern California, people are really into their cars. But you won't keep a BMW or a Mercedes or an Audi as long as you keep your teeth.

YOU ALWAYS WEAR YOUR SMILE. AND IT NEVER GOES OUT OF STYLE

Justene:
I think it's the best return on investment. You always wear your smile.

Janice:
You always wear your smile. And it never goes out of style.

Aurora:
It never goes out of style, that's true.

In some professions, you could probably calculate the return on investment. A salesperson who doesn't smile because they're self-conscious about their teeth, versus someone who has a big, beautiful smile.

Justene:
Most of the successful sales reps that I've met have a really nice smile. Whether it's a veneer, whether it's whitening or Invisalign®, they each have something that enhances their smile.

Janice:

Yes.

Aurora:

We take our teeth for granted. But we know we need to take care of our car. We need to change the tires. The tires won't last forever. We need to change the oil. The engine won't last forever. People take care of their cars. Or the car stops working. That makes sense.

You are making me realize that I've been taking better care of my Mercedes than my teeth. I can get a new car, but I can't get another mouth.

Janice:

Right.

Aurora:

What could be more valuable than a smile that you wear forever?

> YOU ARE MAKING ME REALIZE THAT I'VE BEEN TAKING BETTER CARE OF MY MERCEDES THAN MY TEETH

Or don't wear forever. When I lived in Indonesia, I saw a lot of old people who didn't have many teeth. Just a couple of teeth were left. I don't see that so much in North America, but they might have dentures. It's less obvious.

Janice:

Comparing it to the car is the right way to compare it. It definitely needs maintenance. When you're younger, the car is new. As you get older, it needs more maintenance.

Aurora:

I would love to have you paint a picture, so I understand. Let's take an imaginary person who is 30 who does very proactive "car maintenance" on their teeth. How are they when they're 60?

Justene:

Their quality of life is totally different. Let's say somebody in their 30s has good habits. Brushing twice a day, flossing once a day is a habit. It takes probably between 5 or 10 minutes a day. Staying with it is the key. Be consistent. Have the habit of going to the dentist twice a year for a checkup, cleaning, and regular maintenance.

Someone who develops good habits at age 30 will have good oral health at age 60. For example, I have patients in their 80s, and they have all their real teeth.

Aurora:

Awesome.

Justene:

They tend to be more relaxed and enjoy life more. They don't have to take their teeth out. I can assure you they are a lot less cranky than their counterparts in their 60s who have false teeth.

Janice:

That's for sure.

Justene:

I have patients in their 80s, and they have a full set of teeth, maybe not the whitest color, but they have their own teeth. And they have good habits. They're healthier as well. They don't have as many health issues. Their body doesn't have inflammation caused by plaque building up on their teeth. Overall, they take less medication and are a lot healthier.

Aurora:

What would you see in the case of the 30-year-old with bad habits?

Justene:

They see their dentist every few years, rather than twice every year. They are flossing occasionally versus flossing daily. Consistency is definitely the key to good habits. This 30-year-old may start to experience problems.

But starting in their 40s, they're going to experience problems such as the need for root canals and crowns. Sometimes they get a toothache.

When pain happens, it never happens at a convenient time. Usually it's a holiday like July 4 weekend, or Memorial Day, or Thanksgiving. I get a lot of emergency calls on holidays.

Aurora:

Some big event—like your daughter is getting married.

Justene:

Right. Or graduation. Or you're on a cruise. I've had many people who were on a cruise that docked in San Diego, and we fixed their problem.

Aurora:

So don't want to wait until it's urgent and important.

Justene:

Yes, be proactive.

Aurora:

Take care of your teeth when it's important and not urgent.

Justene:

Starting at the age of 30, I see patients with bad habits experience more problems. They end up spending a lot more money over their 40s and 50s. And they are not spending money on enhancing, but rather fixing a problem they absolutely must fix.

Aurora:

So overall, they are spending more even though they thought they were saving by not going to the dentist every six months.

Janice:

That's right. On average, people spend about $650 by going to see a dentist regularly, according to a 2014 report from the American Dental Association.

On the other hand, people who don't go to see a dentist regularly, can spend $3,000 or more. So, the truth is that you're spending more money by not going to see a dentist on a regular basis.

Justene:

By the time you get to 60, you will definitely lose many teeth—not just one—if you don't have good habits in your 30s, 40s, and 50s.

By the time people get to 60, a lot of them are motivated to get their teeth fixed. Without a lifetime of good habits, they typically have multiple missing teeth by now. They generally eat on one side and not the other.

Janice:

When they start having problems with the one good side, they are out of places to eat.

Justene:

By that time, most people are very motivated to do something about it. And some people can. And some people come a little too late to have good options.

Aurora:

It must weigh on your heart when you see those 60-year-olds who are motivated. If only they had been motivated when they were 50 or 40.

Justene:

That would be so much easier! We love to help patients in their 40s and 50s reclaim their health, confidence, and smile. At 60, you still have options, even if you have neglected your teeth. We can do something about it. It's just not ideal.

7 Secrets to Feeling 7 Years Younger

Aurora:

I'd like to learn more about the keys to a healthy smile after 40. How can people rejuvenate their smiles and feel more youthful, confident and vital? I understand you have 7 secrets to feeling 7 years younger. What is key number one?

Justene:

Having a healthy, happy life is the most important thing. That's our belief and so secret number one is to be free.

KEY #1. BE FREE!

And here, be free means to be free of cavities and gum infection. It's fundamental to good health—but a lot of people don't think about it.

People assume that they will have symptoms if they have cavities or gum infection, but that's a myth. A lot of people don't have symptoms right away. By the time they have symptoms, their situation is much worse.

Cavities and gum infection cause inflammation. Inflammation accelerates aging.

Aurora:
How does inflammation accelerate aging?

Justene:
Inflammation affects your overall health. So, when you have a gum infection, the irritation is not confined to your mouth. You will have inflammation in your body—in your blood vessels, your skin, and more. Inflammation taxes your immune system.

Janice:
Diseases are all related systemically. If you don't have your health under control, then there will be signs and symptoms inside your mouth.

Aurora:
That reminds me of the saying, "Don't look a gift horse in the mouth." Is it true that the mouth reveals age and health? Can you tell the health of a person from their mouth?

Janice:

Many people don't realize that their dentist could save their life. Every year, about 50,000 Americas are diagnosed with oral or throat cancer, according to the American Cancer Society. When detected in the early stages, there is an excellent survival rate of approximately 80-90 percent. We can detect these early signs and symptoms in just a few minutes, and this early detection can save lives.

When we look in your mouth, we can see that inflammation and how it affects your overall health. Everything in the body is connected. Usually bones are hidden inside the body—except for the mouth. That's the only place we can see bones without taking an MRI or CT scan. Your mouth reveals a lot about your overall health.

For example, with sleep apnea, people struggle while they're sleeping. They don't get enough oxygen, so they don't get a deep rest at night. When we look inside the mouth of a person suffering from sleep apnea, we can see the evidence.

Aurora:

Is there a correlation between sleep apnea and unhealthy mouth?

Janice:

Yes, absolutely.

Here's another example: if a person has a narrow arch, they cannot breathe as easily, so they're more likely to have less saliva in their mouth, which makes them prone to cavities and gum infections. That, in turn, makes them more likely to have high blood pressure later.

Aurora:

So secret number one is: be free. What's secret number two to reversing aging?

KEY #2. YOUR TEETH ARE THE FOUNDATION OF YOUR BEAUTY

Janice:

Key number two is your teeth are the foundation of your beauty.

It makes me mad that people over 40 think that the best way to rejuvenate their face is to get plastic surgery. That is just wrong. I'm here today to tell you that the best way to rejuvenate your face is to see a dentist. [See video with diagram here: www.KeysToAHealthySmile.com.]

Did you know that your jawbone is the foundation to your face? No matter how much makeup you put on, or how much plastic surgery you have done, if you don't have a good stable foundation to your face, your face will cave in.

I want to show you a diagram that will help to demonstrate my point. Look at this shocking picture. At the top is a woman with all of her teeth, and because she has her teeth, her bone is intact, and that supports her face.

The middle picture shows a picture of a woman who has lost her back teeth, and because she has lost her back teeth, her bone is melting, and her face is sinking.

The bottom picture shows a woman who has lost all of her teeth. You don't want this. Without the underlying structure of teeth, her jaw bone is melting away. You can see that her face has caved in, and she looks ancient.

My team and I can help people avoid this tragic result. It's what we do at A+ Family

Dentistry. It is possible to reverse the signs of aging by taking proper care of your teeth.

Aurora:

If you don't take care of your teeth, your face is like a house that has termites. Eventually, it crumbles as there is no structural strength underneath the surface.

Justene:

Exactly.

Aurora:

What is secret number three?

Janice:

Secret number three is white teeth make you look younger and more attractive.

KEY #3. WHITE TEETH MAKE YOU LOOK YOUNGER

Janice:

A lot of our patients come in and have a simple whitening procedure. They feel better about their smile, so they smile more. As a result, they're more likely to be sociable at work, to be confident talking, smiling, and connecting with others. Therefore, they often advance in their career and make more money.

There was an interesting study done by the University of Pittsburgh which revealed that people who are smiling are deemed to be more trustworthy than people who are frowning or have a neutral expression. You can see that people who are seen as trustworthy are more likely to get promoted and be more successful overall.

Aurora:
I can see how a confident smile would have a domino effect.

Justene:
USA Today reported that more than half of the top 100 billionaires started out working at another company. The most common first job of the people on Forbes magazine's World Billionaires list was as a salesperson. Successful salespeople have winning smiles.

Aurora:
A winning smile is the first step to closing the sale.

Justene:

As we age, our teeth gradually get yellower. It's such a slow process that we don't notice it. It makes a huge difference to whiten your teeth. It takes years off instantly.

Aurora:

I remember my mom loved tea. She was Canadian, of British descent, so she was a big tea drinker. Over time, the tea stained her teeth. You're right, it did make her look older.

Justene:

Red wine and coffee will also stain teeth. It's easy to whiten teeth, and our patients are amazed how much younger they look.

Aurora:

These are good secrets to reducing aging by seven years. What's secret number four?

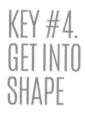

KEY #4.
GET INTO
SHAPE

Justene:

Key number four is to get into shape. Get your body—and your teeth—into good shape.

Janice:

Focus on eating better, exercising, and taking care of your health. And get in shape with your teeth.

You use your teeth every day for 40 years, so eventually, they wear down. As you age, your teeth get shorter, and you look older.

When you compare photographs, you'll notice that your smile is not as big and bright as it once was. So you look older.

Aurora:

I never really thought about that, but it makes sense. Your teeth are going to get shorter. How much do you lose? It must be very small, but it's still perceptible.

Janice:

Right.

Justene:

Everyone is a little bit different. Some people wear down their teeth significantly, and they have no idea.

You'd be surprised, Aurora, but you can compare before and after pictures. I'd say between 40% to 60% of people over 40 have worn their teeth down significantly.

Janice:

Mm-hmm (affirmative).

Justene:

We get into our 40s, and many people begin to have what we call a reverse smile. Do you know what a reverse smile is?

Aurora:

No, what's a reverse smile?

Justene:

So, you know like when we smile, it's like a like a curve. But—when people wear down their front teeth, their smile goes upside down. Like a frown.

Janice:

It's a reverse smile.

Justene:

Their four front teeth wear down significantly, so when they smile, it almost looks like a frown. It's very distracting, but the patient doesn't realize that because it happens so gradually over time. They don't notice how it dramatically changes their smile and their face.

Aurora:

Wow. And you can rectify that?

Janice:

Yes, we can fix that.

Justene:

So, that's what we mean by: get into shape.

Justene:

To summarize, there are two elements to getting your teeth into shape. First, there's the reverse smile—the smile that's like a frown—due to the front teeth wearing down significantly over time.

Second, many older patients have irregular teeth, often chipped from wear. It distracts from their smile.

Naturally, your eye is drawn to whatever is not in harmony with their face. But when you talk to a person, you want to look them in the eye, and not be distracted by their teeth.

Janice:

You can be destroying your teeth without even knowing it. If you don't get your teeth into shape, it is much more likely that you will lose a tooth or two.

Your teeth are like an M&M candy. It's hard on the outside, so that's like your enamel, but once you break that shell, the chocolate underneath melts easily. It is softer.

So once the hard outer enamel no longer protects your teeth, they start eroding faster and faster.

Getting into shape is not only cosmetic. It's also functional and structural. The shape of your teeth impacts the mechanics of chewing. As you get older, your teeth wear down. The chewing system can become out of balance.

Aurora:

Do you recommend braces for people over 40?

Janice:

Yes—Justene has braces right now.

Aurora:

Right, I'm looking at somebody with braces!

Janice:

The Invisalign® are barely visible.

Aurora:

What's secret number 5?

Janice:

So, number five is to use protection at night.

Aurora:

That's cute.

KEY #5. USE PROTECTION AT NIGHT

Janice:

In dentistry, that's considered your night guard or your retainer. Wearing a night guard can help protect your teeth while you're sleeping.

I ask new patients, do you grind your teeth at night? They often say no, I'm fine.

Then I see them again five years later, and the difference is shocking. They have worn out their teeth! They don't even realize how they're doing it. The problem is that they are grinding their teeth at night.

Aurora:

Do you recommend a night guard for everyone? Or only for people who are grinding their teeth?

Justene:

The majority of patients benefit from using a night guard for a few months after we put their teeth into the correct bite position. It depends on what we see, and if they are taking any medication.

Grinding and clenching can be triggered by medication. There's a lot of medication in our society nowadays. Most people don't know that it can trigger grinding.

Aurora:
Anything else?

Justene:
If I had worn my retainer, I wouldn't have to get braces put on again after 40. So let that be a warning to others to follow their dentist's instructions the first time. Use protection at night. By that we mean, wear your night guard or retainer.

Aurora:
The voice of experience. What is secret number six that can help people rejuvenate?

KEY #6.
HEALTHY DIET, HEALTHY TEETH

Janice:
Secret number six is that a healthy diet creates a healthy smile. Avoid acidic or sug-

140

ary food or drinks to keep your teeth healthy and strong.

A lot of time, people don't realize that food and drink can wear away your teeth. Even just the vinegar in your salad or sugary sodas will damage your teeth. You will melt away the enamel. And once it's lost, we cannot put it back. Even when we put it back with porcelain or something stronger, it's not the same as your natural enamel. So our job is to help you keep it—so we need your help to maintain it and not wear it away.

Aurora:

Even vinegar is bad?

Janice:

A little is fine, but over the years, it does add up.

Aurora:

Over many decades, your habits impact your health and your teeth.

Justene:

Soda pop and even sports drinks or energy drinks are terrible. There is so much sugar in those drinks!

Aurora:

Do you think sugar is the main culprit?

Justene:

Yes, we recommend cutting out sugar. The worst thing we see is when people bathe their teeth in sugar, by sipping soda or energy drinks all day long.

Janice:

High sugar content can occur in things we think are healthy—like coconut water or orange juice.

Justene:

Eat foods that are more alkaline on the pH scale. Some everyday foods like bread, corn, coffee, milk, alcohol, meat, are all more acidic. Vegetables are more alkaline.

Janice:

Healthy diet, healthy teeth!

Aurora:

Alright, let's have the final secret to feeling seven years younger.

Drum roll, please!

Justene:

This one is cute. Go for it, Janice.

Janice:

The last secret that we want to share is—smile! Smiling helps you feel more confident and look younger. Your smile is the sexiest curve on your body!

Justene:

And everyone knows how to do it. Even when you're having a bad day, if you force yourself to smile, pretty soon, your day will turn around. Not only does your smile communicate how you're feeling—it affects how you are feeling.

In one study, participants were forced to smile by holding chopsticks in their mouths. Even though their smiles were forced, the result was the participants bounced back faster from stress, as reported in Psychological Science.

Aurora:

Thich Nhat Hanh said, "Sometimes your joy is the source of your smile, but sometimes your smile can be the source of your joy."

Janice:

Exactly. Not only does smiling make you feel good, it also makes other people feel good. Smiling is contagious. If you smile, pretty soon the people around you are smiling back at you.

Justene:

Smiling may even strengthen your body on a cellular level, according to biochemist Sondra Barrett, author of "Secrets of Your Cells." Smiling may release tension on the cellular level, as well.

Janice:

It feels good, it's good for you, and it's free. So smile!

Justene:

To recap, the 7 keys to feeling 7 years younger are:

1. Be Free

2. Your Teeth are the Foundation of Your Beauty

3. White Teeth Make You Look Younger

4. Get into Shape

5. Use Protection at Night

6. Healthy Diet, Healthy Teeth

7. Smile!

FAQ

Aurora:

What else should people know about oral health as they age? Let's cover some of the most frequently-asked questions.

Justene:

A lot of our patients in the 50-year-old-range start thinking it's too late. Some of them are embarrassed, because they know they neglected their health during their 40s. Whether because of their career or family, they do feel embarrassed.

My advice is that you still have a lot of options. So just come on in. Let us help you before you get to the point of having no good options. It's time for you to take care of yourself. It's not too late at all. That's my advice to people in their 50s.

Aurora:

I've been feeling embarrassed that I haven't gone to the dentist quarterly, not even close. I realize now, talking to you both, that I should have been more proactive.

But you two are so accepting and kind. Not a bit of scolding or fault-finding. Instead, exploring options for what can be done, starting now. That's a lovely gift that you give to others.

IT'S NOT YOUR FAULT. DENTISTS HAVEN'T DONE A GOOD JOB OF EDUCATING THE PUBLIC

Justene:

Thanks. It's not your fault. Dentists haven't done a good job of educating the public on different issues or how to have optimal oral health. This is our profession. Whether it's our inability or our unwillingness to communicate to our patients at large, many people don't have the information they need. It's not your fault.

Aurora:

It's great that you're spreading the message now. I was amazed to learn that daily flossing was one of two things associated with longevity. So floss for a long healthy

life. I've always had good habits with flossing and brushing my teeth. But I didn't see a
dentist semi-annually.

Justene:

Yes, but you could change your mind with
the right information. Once you realize, and
you see the logic behind it, you can change
your mind in an instant.

Aurora:

I already have changed my mind, thanks
to you two.

Justene:

You change your mind, you change your
habits. It's not that hard.

Aurora:

I'm grateful to you because I'm seeing how
important it is to take care of my teeth and
the value of seeing a dentist sooner rather
than later. Even though it can be expensive
or time-consuming, and that's why I have
sometimes procrastinated.

But the metaphor of maintaining a car, that
makes good sense. If you don't take good

care of your car, pretty soon you're driving a beater when you could have a nice car.

Justene:

And by the end, you're going to have to spend a lot more money to fix up that car. Regular maintenance is cheaper overall.

With a car, you can always buy a new one. With your teeth, you can't get another set.

Aurora:

Right. People are living healthy lives longer and longer. It didn't matter so much when people had an average life expectancy of 45, but now it's possible to be vibrant and vital at 60, at 70, at 80, at 90.

Justene:

Totally.

Aurora:

Getting your message out about dental care and proactive health is important. If we don't dramatically change how we think about caring for our teeth, our bodies will have the potential of living longer, but our unhealthy mouth will sabotage our overall health.

Justene:

True. The health of your mouth or your oral health is definitely linked to your overall or systemic health. If you're healthy and don't have a lot of inflammation in your mouth, that would translate to a lot fewer problems in your overall health.

When you have a lot of bacteria in your mouth from gum disease—from gingivitis or gum infection or cavities—it increases the inflammation in your mouth and your body significantly.

That inflammation is linked to a 40% to 60% higher risk of stroke or heart attack.

Janice:

Poor oral health significantly increases the risk of having a stroke or heart attack.

POOR ORAL HEALTH INCREASES THE RISK OF HAVING A STROKE OR HEART ATTACK

Justene:

If you have gingivitis or a gum problem, it can increase your risk of having a stroke or heart attack by 40% to 60%.

Aurora:

That's huge.

Justene:

Absolutely. We receive requests for medical clearances all the time for patients who are going to have through knee replacement or hip replacement. We have to confirm that they have a healthy mouth.

Aurora:

Because they're not healthy enough for a knee or hip replacement?

Justene:

Exactly. Then afterward, they're not supposed to have any dental work for another four months. So if a tooth is about to break, they would have to receive dental care first. Poor oral health can jeopardize your chances for other medical care.

Aurora:

I think very few people understand that. As I mentioned last night over dinner, after my father had a heart attack, he had to wait to have bypass surgery. He had to get his wisdom teeth out first. That's not something you want to do right after you've had a heart attack and before major surgery!

Justene:

Most people don't share that story. So people don't know that can be a problem until it happens to them.

Aurora:

It's up to you two to spread the message.

Justene:

Yes, it's better not to have dental surgery and heart surgery at the same time, especially as people age.

Aurora:

What else is important as people age?

Janice:

When you're younger, say 20 or 30, you had fillings done. Some of these can wear out, or they can leak, and then you can get decay in the tooth underneath the old filling. Be proactive coming back to the dentist when you're 40.

We take X-rays so we can see what's underneath. We can take preventative measures and replace old fillings earlier, which can save the tooth underneath. Being proactive can mean be the difference between simply replacing that filling, versus needing a crown, or losing the tooth altogether.

Aurora:
Goodbye tooth.

Janice:
Early intervention is key.

EARLY INTERVENTION IS KEY

Aurora:
"An ounce of prevention is worth a pound of cure" as the saying goes.

Janice:
Yes. Some people think everything is OK, because they don't feel any pain. But, if you have had a root canal already, that means the nerve has been taken out already. So your body cannot tell you if something is wrong.

There's no alarm system going on saying, "I have an infection" or "Oh, I should take care of this." There's no alarm system anymore.

Aurora:

So a root canal removes the nerve and removes the pain signal. Can you have a root canal for just one tooth?

Janice:

Yes.

Justene:

So then you don't have sensation for that one tooth.

Janice:

Then you don't feel pain. But pain tells us there's a problem.

Justene:

Also, we have patients who are on pain medication for various reasons, such as back pain or shoulder pain or arthritis. And that masks a toothache as well. Patients on pain medication don't feel a toothache either. Again, regular exams twice a year are helpful, so you could discover these problems and take care of them.

Aurora:

So they might not be aware there's a problem, and meanwhile, they could be getting to the point of no return.

Justene:

Correct.

Janice:

Some people focus on the wrong problem or issue. I have patients that have missing teeth, and they look older than their age. Instead of fixing their teeth to rejuvenate their face, they get plastic surgery.

Justene:

Your teeth and your jaw bone are the foundation of your face. People would be wise to consider taking care of their teeth before they get plastic surgery, as we mentioned in the 7 keys to feeling 7 years younger.

Janice:

Typically, plastic surgeons are not educated about dentistry. Teeth are not their area of expertise, so they don't know. They're trying to make the face look better; but they cannot create an optimal result without the right foundation.

Justene:

Unfortunately, there's a disconnect between dentists and plastic surgeons.

Aurora:

In other words, your face is like a house built on a concrete foundation. Your teeth and jaw are that solid foundation.

So they're in there doing the interior decorating, changing the paint color, changing the kitchen cabinets, but if there's no foundation holding up the house, it's going to go down in the next mudslide. Is that about right?

Justene:

Yes, you got it.

Janice:

Some people keep going to their plastic surgeon to do more work and more work, but it's still the same result.

Aurora:

Right, because they don't have the foundation. It makes sense, once you think about it.

Let's define a few simple terms to make sure everyone is on the same page. Dentistry 101: What is a root canal?

WHAT IS A ROOT CANAL?

Justene:

There's a nerve in the middle of the tooth. When you get a cavity, and it gets to the nerve, that's when you feel pain.

So, a root canal is a dental procedure that removes the cavity and the infected nerve. The doctor puts a filling down your roots. So the tooth stays there.

Aurora:

The tooth is there, but it's dead?

Justene:

Yes, so functionally, you still have a tooth. That way, you don't lose your foundation.

Aurora:

I see.

Justene:

But then if you get a cavity later on, you're not going to feel any pain. Basically, the alarm system is turned off on that tooth.

Janice:

That's called a root canal.

Justene:

After the root canal, we put a crown on top to replace the missing pieces of the tooth, and it looks very natural. It's strong. You can eat normally. You can smile normally. You still have to regularly check to make sure it's in good condition.

Aurora:

Right now, as you know, I have a temporary crown and I'm getting the permanent one soon. What is the difference between a temporary crown and a permanent one? What are they made of? Are they durable? What can you teach us about crowns?

Justene:

Crowns are an excellent way to preserve the tooth structure that was lost, either due to a cavity or a fracture. In your case, it was a fracture. Temporary crowns are not plastic but are made from a plastic-like material. That material is not strong enough or dense enough to seal your tooth permanently.

Your permanent or final crown is made of porcelain. It's very strong. It's aesthetically pleasing. It looks like your natural enamel. It will seal your tooth for a long time. That's the main difference between a temporary and a final crown.

Aurora:

How long does a crown last? 10 years? 20 years?

Justene:

Good question. It depends on your home care habits, and on your bite. A crown could last anywhere between 5 to 30 years.

Aurora:

So it depends on my bite, or a person's bite. Tell me more. Do you mean whether they're grinding their teeth at night?

Janice:

Exactly.

Justene:

Grinding makes a crown wear out faster. Or if the person is not going to the dentist regularly for cleanings every quarter and an annual checkup, then there can be a lot more bacterial plaque around the crown. That could cause a cavity on the underneath tooth structure under the crown, and that would make it defective.

Aurora:
Can people have a bite that is a problem, or is it just grinding at night?

Justene:
Absolutely. People need braces if their teeth are not lined up correctly.

Janice:
That puts more pressure on their teeth, and they can break.

Or people who have one crown, but they don't have any other teeth around it, their bite would be different. When they eat, more force is on that single tooth with the crown, and so the crown will wear out faster with all that pressure.

Aurora:
Again, it's like the foundation of the house. If you have a solid foundation, you're good. But if you take out the other pillars, the one that's left has more pressure on it.

Justene:

As we talk about it, it becomes easy to understand.

Aurora:

It becomes much more straightforward—not such a mysterious thing. The way you explain things, it makes complete sense.

What about wisdom teeth? What do you recommend if somebody is 40 and they still have their wisdom teeth? Or they're 60 and they still have their wisdom teeth? Or they're 80 like my dad?

What are wisdom teeth, first of all, let's start there.

Justene:

Wisdom teeth are the very last molars in your mouth. They're way in the back, in the corner of your jaw.

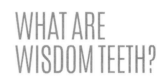

WHAT ARE WISDOM TEETH?

Aurora:

Under what circumstances do you recommend removing wisdom teeth?

Justene:

It depends, as everyone's anatomy is different. The ideal age to check on your wisdom teeth is between 17 to 18 years old. The younger the patient, the easier it is to remove wisdom teeth. Recovery and healing are better and faster.

Sometimes the wisdom teeth come out straight, and if there's enough room in your mouth, then they do not need to be taken out.

But, if there is a potential problem, we recommend having them removed. Most of the time, wisdom teeth don't align properly, so people usually don't use them to eat. Sometimes, they don't come out at all.

Aurora:

If you have somebody who is 60 and they haven't had their wisdom teeth out yet, would you still recommend removing them?

Justene:

If they needed to. If they have a cavity that we cannot reach to fill, or if the cavity is so big that it requires a root canal.

Aurora:

(laughs)
Open wide! Even wider.

Janice:

(laughs)

Can I take your lower jaw out?

Aurora:

With wisdom teeth, do you recommend doing one half then the other half, or the whole mouth at one time?

Justene:

Normally, it is easiest to have done all at once.

Aurora:

Do you recommend antibiotics?

Justene:

It depends. Everyone is different.

Aurora:

It's not one size fits all. You tailor what you recommend to each person.

Justene:

Absolutely.

Janice:

Everyone's immune system is different, their genetics are different, their facial profile is different. How they recover, how they heal, how their teeth line up together, how their teeth relate to their jaw, everyone is different.

Justene:

I haven't seen two patients that are alike.

Janice:

Even when they're related. People are like snowflakes.

Aurora:

What is a veneer?

Justene:

A veneer is a partial crown. It covers the front surface of your teeth. A veneer can be used to change the shape and color of your teeth. Typically, people get four or six front teeth or 10 front teeth done together.

Today, almost all the big movie stars have veneers.

Aurora:

They all have perfect teeth.

Justene:

Veneers are the secret of those megawatt Hollywood smiles.

MEGAWATT HOLLYWOOD

Nicholas Cage, Tom Cruise, Cheryl Cole, Victoria Beckham, Catherine Zeta-Jones, Gwen Stefani, Miley Cyrus and many more movie stars all appear to have massively improved their star power—and their smiles— with veneers.

Veneers used to be aggressive, meaning that we would have to remove a lot of tooth structure to put them on. Now, the material is so much better, so veneers can be much thinner. That means that we have to remove very little tooth structure.

I'm thinking of getting veneers myself. I turned 40 a couple of years ago, so I think it's time for me to treat myself to veneers.

Aurora:

I've been thinking that veneers would be a good idea for me, too. But I worry about what you said. You can't just paint a veneer on top of the tooth. How much of your healthy tooth has to be removed?

Justene:

Previously, we had to remove a millimeter. When you think of a millimeter, it's not a lot, but on teeth, it's a fair amount. Before, dentists would remove about a millimeter of the front surface of the tooth to add a veneer. Nowadays, it's only .3 to .5 of a millimeter. So it's 30% to 50% of what it was previously.

Aurora:

That's a big difference. Does veneer only change the color of the tooth?

Justene:

Yes, and it also changes the shape.

Aurora:

So that's how movie stars get perfectly shaped white teeth.

Justene:

Right.

Aurora:

How long do veneers last?

Justene:

They can last from 5 to 30 years, like a crown. Usually, the front ones last longer because people tend to keep their teeth clean better in the front. If you keep it clean and cavity free, a veneer can last for a long time.

Aurora:

Do veneers need special care?

Justene:

Veneers are made from a glass-like material. They are strong, but not as strong as a healthy tooth. Everyone is different. Some people have a very strong bite, and in that case, we recommend wearing a night guard. It's like a retainer, so people don't put too much pressure on their teeth at night. So there's a little bit of additional care when you have veneers.

Janice:

You're not supposed to bite on an apple or something hard, like a hard candy, as that might break or chip a veneer. But you should treat your teeth the same way, you shouldn't bite on anything hard anyway.

Aurora:

Are veneers more sensitive to hot and cold?

Janice:

No, not really, because you're still on enamel. It might be for the first few days because of the work that we have done. But the veneer shouldn't create temperature sensitivity.

Aurora:

What is the difference between teeth whitening and veneer?

Justene:

Teeth whitening whitens your own natural teeth.

A veneer is something a dentist has to make. We shape the tooth, we send it to the lab, the lab fabricates the thin crown material, then we bond it on.

A veneer is like a permanent whitening. With the additional benefit that you can change the shape at the same time.

Aurora:

Why do you change the shape?

Justene:

Teeth are not exactly symmetrical. A beautiful smile, like a beautiful face, is balanced and symmetrical. So we make everything more balanced and symmetrical.

I remember the first time I whitened my teeth, I was in dental school, and I was 25 at the time. I whitened my teeth once every three or four years, and they stay white. But now as I've turned 40, I feel like I need a touch up every six months.

Janice:

Every three months is ideal for people over 40 who want to maintain white teeth.

Aurora:

So it's like doing the roots for your hair. You need to keep the maintenance going.

Justene:

That's why veneers are so popular.

Aurora:

Do you do a lot of teeth whitening at A+ Family Dentistry?

Janice:

Yes, we do.

Aurora:

What do you recommend to whiten teeth?

Justene:

Zoom® was the standard whitening for a long time. Personally, I don't like Zoom® because it caused my teeth to be sensitive.

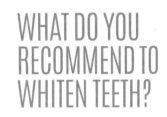

WHAT DO YOU RECOMMEND TO WHITEN TEETH?

Janice:

Everyone's teeth are different. Some have thicker enamel, some have thinner enamel. Some people wear out their teeth more, so they get more sensitive. Some people still have thicker enamel, so it's less sensitive.

Justene:

Now we recommend GLO for whitening. It was developed by Dr. Jonathan B. Levine, a dentist and NYU professor.

I tried it in August of last year for the first time, and I loved it. I didn't have any problem with sensitivity. So now we do a lot of GLO whitening at A+ Family Dentistry.

Aurora:

How long does it take?

Justene:

It usually takes about an hour in our office. It is easy—you're not numb or anything like that. The material is applied to your teeth. You are there for an hour, and your teeth will be significantly whitened—usually five to seven shades whiter in color.

Aurora:

That's a lot whiter!

Justene:

Absolutely. August of last year I did it, so that was five months ago, and now I want to do it again. Coffee, tea, red wine and a few other things stain the teeth. I recommend a regular touch up every six months or so, depending on your diet.

Aurora:

People used to get white spots on their teeth due to fluoride. Do you see that in your patients?

Justene:
We don't see a lot of dental fluorosis or mottled enamel anymore.

Janice:
It's changed because now everywhere in the US we have standardized fluoride in the water. The only time I see spots now is when kids have braces, and they don't take care of their teeth. Once they take off their braces, they sometimes have those spots. But there are medications they can use at home daily that help to reduce that.

Aurora:
What kind of toothbrushes do you recommend?

Justene:
We advocate the electric toothbrush, but not all electric toothbrushes are equal! (laughs)

NOT ALL TOOTHBRUSHES ARE EQUAL

Generally, the battery-powered one, where you have to put in a battery, is not great. The spin electric toothbrush is not great.

We love the Philips Sonicare™ When I was in dental school, I tried Sonicare™, and I didn't like it at that time. The technology was more abrasive early on.

The last two model are excellent: Philips Sonicare™ FlexCare and Diamond Clean. It's ultrasonic technology, so it's similar to when you go into a dental office you get the ultrasonic cleaning. It doesn't cut anything, it just vibrates, and the sound waves break up the tartar build up.

Aurora:
Is it a toothbrush or is it a jet of water?

Justene:
It's an ultrasonic toothbrush. It vibrates at 30,000 strokes per minute.

Janice:
30,000 strokes per minute—you can't do that manually.

Aurora:
I saw those in your office. I want one! (laughs)

Justene:

(laughs)

We'll send you one. There's a right way to use it. It's an excellent tool, but it's a tool. Like any tool, you have to know how to use it the right way. We coach our patients how to use an electronic toothbrush.

Aurora:

What's the right way to use it?

Justene:

So many people use electronic toothbrushes the wrong way. People do it the wrong way on "The Housewives of Beverly Hills."

We have a video on our website to demonstrate the right way. It's much easier to show on a video.

Aurora:

People can watch the video online at www.APlusFamilyDentistry.com.

Justene:

That's the best way.

Janice:

There's another important point about toothbrushes. A lot of people use a manual toothbrush with a medium or hard bristle.

They don't realize that it's damaging their gums and teeth. They wear down more of their gums and enamel. But they feel clean, and they're used to that. So, if they switch to a soft bristle toothbrush, they use it for maybe a week, then they return to their old habits.

Aurora:

I'm glad that you brought that up. I'm one of those "I love brushing my teeth" people.

You're exactly right. I would use the soft bristle for a little while, then go back to the medium bristle as it seemed to be getting my teeth cleaner. But now I'm paying the price because my gums are receding. So you're giving great advice. Listen to this at home, kids!

(laughs)

Justene:

One day at a time people don't see the full consequences. It's a myth that a hard bristle is better than a soft bristle.

Dangerous Dental Myths

Janice:

There are different myths in dentistry. I don't think that dentists are doing an adequate job educating patients.

Aurora:

What are some dangerous dental myths?

Janice:

One myth is that if you lose a tooth, it's okay. But the truth is that losing a tooth is not okay.

It's like your analogy of caring for your car. Imagine you are driving your car. Instead of four wheels, it only has only three wheels.

People think they can eat on the other side of their mouth, but they would never continue to drive a car with a missing wheel. They would fix it.

Aurora:

True. What other myths are there?

Justene:

I think gum infection is under-diagnosed by some dentists. Often, treating gum disease is not covered by insurance because it has been there for a long time. Some dentists give up recommending treating it because insurance doesn't cover it.

The right thing to do is to take the time to explain to the patient why they need it and give the patient a chance to pay for the service if it is not covered by insurance. I see some dentists doing regular cleaning—which is above the gum—and not treating the infection underneath the gum.

It is important to recommend what is best for the patient and take the time to explain things.

Aurora:

What about mercury fillings? Are they okay, or is that another myth?

Janice:

With metal fillings, if they don't cause any problems, if they don't have any cracks, then the patient can keep them longer.

But personally, I replaced all of my metal fillings, and Justene did as well, because we believe in optimal health. When you chew, mercury fillings create mercury vapor. Then you breathe in that mercury vapor, you inhale that through your body. Personally, I think that it's best to replace them. But I know some other dentists don't agree with that.

Aurora:
Do you remove mercury fillings in your office?

Justene:
Yes, we use high-speed suction to get the vapor out as we remove the mercury fillings.

Aurora:
What other myths are there?

Janice:
There's a myth that fluoride treatment is bad for kids. The truth is that fluoride treatment is good for kids.

A lot of parents are worried about fluoride treatment because they've read online that it's bad for them. But you can't believe everything you read on the internet. So these parents don't want their kids to have fluoride treatment after their cleanings so, therefore, their kids get more cavities.

Justene:
Fluoride is toxic in high concentration, but I don't believe that it's a problem in low concentration.

Janice:
I use it on my son. If it were toxic, I wouldn't use it.

Aurora:
You use it on your precious son, who is two years old, right?

Janice:
Yes.

Aurora:
Then you would obviously recommend it to your patients. Are there any other myths that you would like to share?

Justene:
Myth: You can use mouthwash instead of flossing.

Fact: People need to floss.

Aurora:
Do you think mouthwash is to be avoided or is it benign?

Janice:
It's okay to use in conjunction or in addition to brushing and flossing, but it's not a replacement.

Oil pulling is a myth.

Aurora:
What is oil pulling?

Justene:
Oil pulling is a new trend on Facebook and the internet.
(laughs)

Aurora:
Okay, that's a reputable source.
(laughs)

Justene:
Oil pulling is holding coconut oil in your mouth for two minutes.

Myth: Oil pulling treats gum infection.

Fact: It doesn't.

Aurora:
I heard hydrogen peroxide does something similar.

Justene:
It helps, but it doesn't replace proper care.

Aurora:
Is coconut oil helpful? Or not at all?

Justene:
It's a little bit helpful, like adjunctive, like in addition to, but people think that it replaces proper habits altogether.

Aurora:
Is it ever too late to see a dentist?

I'm interested in longevity. Say you have a new patient who is 70, and you look at their teeth and you see that they could benefit from having their wisdom teeth out, would you still recommend it at 70? Or would you say that it's too late?

IS IT EVER TOO LATE TO SEE A DENTIST?

Justene:

Our philosophy is: never give up.

But we don't put patients through torture either. I have a few patients in my practice who can't take care of themselves anymore, but a cleaning is still helpful. We recommend every two months or even once a month if they can't brush their teeth anymore.

That's going to reduce the amount of pain in their body. When food gets stuck, it can be painful. We have a few patients where we do cleaning and not a whole lot of dental work, just to maintain their general cleanliness for them. And to boost their self-esteem.

Aurora:

Your point about self-esteem is not minor.

My grandmother, for example, was a school teacher. She was quick and clever. She never used a calculator, she did math in her head. Super smart, definitely the alpha in that family.

She was a little bitty thing, maybe 110 pounds, if that. She was always slender. She wore a corset. She didn't need to wear a corset. She always wore a dress; she always wore shoes with a little heel. She looked ready to play the piano at her church every day.

I think her rules about how she showed up in the world added a great deal of value to her life. She dressed smart; she was smart. She was confident in her own demure way.

Life can be challenging. In my grandmother's case, her husband died young.

People struggle in the aftermath of death, divorce or disease. But if you feel good about yourself, you can bounce back more quickly, be more resilient.

Studies show that happy people live seven years longer, are 35% less likely to get sick, and earn a million dollars more over their lifetime, according to Dr. Edward Diener, the author of "Happiness."

Self-esteem is an asset. It's not a trivial thing to feel better about yourself, in my experience. Tell me about some of your patients. Do you help transform their self-esteem?

Patient Success Stories

Justene:

Absolutely. I've seen patients arrive at our offices with low self-esteem, and then leave with high self-esteem, and it seems like they are two different people. They're so much happier.

Aurora:

People are helpful to smiling, confident people.

Let's talk about vanity. As a Leo, I have a lot of expertise in that area.
(laughs).

What about people who want to get their teeth whitened, what do you recommend?

Justene:

Recently, we had a patient in her early 30s. She hadn't had a date for the last five years because of her two front teeth.

Aurora:
That's a big price to pay, not dating.

Janice:
Especially in her early 30s.

Justene:
Her front teeth were not attractive. She hadn't dated for five to six years, and she hated it. She was very grumpy when she came in.

Aurora:
I guess so.

Justene:
She told us that. She was concerned about the cost, and she was a bit apprehensive about dental care in general. But it was easy to give her a pretty smile. We fixed her front teeth in just two appointments, two weeks apart.

She loved the result. She was transformed—a lot happier and more pleasant. She wasn't the type to jump up and hug us, but she was clearly thrilled. Quite the contrast from the grumpy young woman we met initially. And it was a very simple fix for us. Seeing her smiling and happy was so rewarding for me.

Aurora:

You got her back in the dating game. I hope she invites you to the wedding.

Justene:

We have many patients in their 60s who start dating again. Sometimes they're finally retired and have more time to enjoy their life, including dating. We help them by restoring or rehabilitating their smile.

Quite a few patients in their 60s are missing a few teeth, or have broken teeth. They come to us and want to fix their teeth.

Sometimes we can take their smile to perfect, and sometimes it's not perfect, but still vastly improved.

It's a joy to watch people transform as their smile improves over a month or two. Usually, they arrive with longer hair, maybe a bushy beard hiding their teeth, and baggy clothes, as if they are trying to be invisible.

As we work on improving their smile, people get their hair cut, their beard trimmed. Pretty soon they have new clothes that fit well. They have confident smiles and are ready to greet the world.

Janice:

Big transformation!

Justene:

It's so rewarding to see them happy. It's so satisfying.

Janice:

It is. I had a patient call me right after her daughter's wedding. She had veneers that had been there for more than ten years, and one of them had chipped. So she came in wanting to fix that.

As she was going through the pictures of her daughter's wedding, she noticed her smile had faded. She was about 50 years old. She didn't like how her teeth looked; she didn't like how she looked. She asked us what she could do.

I recommended new veneers, as her old ones had worn out and changed color over time. She agreed.

So we did new veneers for her, and she was thrilled. She has a beautiful smile again.

She told us that she wanted to redo the photos with my daughter for her wedding. So now she is getting new pictures taken with her daughter.

I had another patient that had a crooked tooth, and he was so embarrassed. He was young, only in his mid-30s. He would not smile.

He was single. He tried to talk to the ladies, but he lacked confidence. He was convinced that people were concentrating on his crooked front tooth.

Aurora:
He was self-conscious.

Janice:
I asked him, "What would you like to change about your smile?"

He said, "I want whiter teeth, I want this tooth to be straighter."

He was relieved that I asked him what he wanted. He said no one had ever talked to him about fixing the tooth that had caused him so much embarrassment.

I gave him what he requested, and now he's happy. He had avoided being in photos before, but now he takes selfies! So he's much more confident. He has started dating.

Aurora:

You seek to understand exactly what your patients need and want.

A plastic surgeon named Maxwell Maltz wrote an excellent book, "Psycho-Cybernetics." Maxwell Maltz became fascinated with self-image and psychology. He noticed dramatic shifts after some people had plastic surgery, but not in other cases.

For example, if someone was troubled by the way their nose looked, and he fixed their nose, their whole personality would change. Their income would improve, their love life would improve, their self-confidence would improve.

In other cases, he would give a patient a beautiful nose, but their self-image wouldn't shift. Their lives and outlook would not change. They would continue to see themselves as ugly, in spite of contrary evidence in the mirror.

Dr. Maltz wanted to understand what made the difference. He discovered the power of self-image. The way his patients thought about their identity was what made the difference between failure and success. Sometimes he would just talk to his patients and help them shift their identity, and their lives would be transformed without any plastic surgery.

So he realized that for optimal results, it was essential to deal with the whole person—body, mind, and spirit—and not just the body.

I see that is what you're doing. You are both healers. You care about people; you're broadcasting unconditional love. It's impossible to be around you without being uplifted by your positive outlook on life.

There's something magical about the two of you, and I think that's it—that's your secret sauce. What do you think?

Janice:
I think you have a point. We listen deeply. We care. We give our patients the opportunity to express their concerns and desires.

We don't just solve the problem. When we recommend a solution, we walk them through the process. We let them know what result to expect after the procedure, and how it can enhance their life.

We show them a mockup of how it will look, and ask what they like about it, and what they don't like about it. That way, they are involved. We explain that we can change this and make you more feminine, or we can make this longer and give you a different look. What is it that you're looking for?

So our patients are engaged with the process and share what they want, and what they like about themselves.

Aurora:

See, you are like Dr. Maltz, dealing with the whole person—body, mind, and spirit—and not just the body. It's so important for people to be heard and understood. It's important to tailor your solution to meet their preferences.

Your process also helps them visualize themselves transformed, both inside and out.

Janice:

Right, there is a transformation within. Having a beautiful smile is not just about health or vanity. It's also about how they feel, their self-confidence, their self-esteem.

Justene:

Melanie Greene is another patient that we had the pleasure of helping.

She's small and frail, in her mid-60s. When she came to us, she had terrible teeth. She also had cancer at the time and was going through treatment. I'm not sure if it was because of the cancer treatment, or because of many years of neglect, but she was having a lot of problems.

She had cavities everywhere. So we treated her.

We started with her top teeth. All 12 of them needed attention—root canals and crowns. We got her top teeth in good shape.

But then her health turned for the worse. During this time, we accommodated her schedule. We would schedule a two-hour appointment, but if she wasn't feeling well, then we would have to reschedule. We saw her every few months.

Janice:

She started losing her hair, she got skinnier, she couldn't eat much. Her food had to go in the blender, like baby food. She wasn't enjoying her liquid diet.

Justene:

But the good thing is that we saved her top teeth. We started just in the nick of time. Otherwise, she would have lost a lot more of her top teeth.

She came back after being away for three or four months. But by this time, she had lost four front teeth on the bottom, and she had many cavities in her remaining teeth. It was so bad that she had to go to hospital to have her teeth surgically removed.

Aurora:

So a few months can make a big difference. Cancer must have decimated her health.

Justene:

Yes. She came in again after she got better in three or four months. She wanted some lower front teeth. She was still fighting for her well-being.

Aurora:

Good for her. Spunky.

Justene:

She appreciated having us on her team. Even if she was going to lose her battle with cancer in a month, she was determined to fight it. She came in and said, "I want some front teeth."

Janice:

It was difficult dental work because she couldn't open her mouth very wide.

Justene:

We were along her side, fighting her battle with her and keeping things going. As Churchill said, "Never, never, never give up."

Aurora:

That's so important. Once you give up, you begin to die.

Justene:

Now all her teeth are fixed. Patients like Melanie Greene make our day.

Aurora:

Spending the last two days interviewing you has been an enlightening experience for me. I hope that people who read this book have this same experience. I went from thinking that dentistry is mysterious and slightly dangerous to realizing that it makes common sense.

You lifted the veil with information and kindness, so there's not a kick of embarrassment that I didn't know—or didn't act on—this information earlier. I feel empowered that it's not too late. There are so many things that can be done.

Thanks to you, I understand how important it is to have a healthy mouth to avoid disease—like a heart attack or stroke.

I learned how much a healthy smile boosts self-confidence, and how much that matters for a sense of well-being.

I learned that keeping your teeth is essential to keeping your jawbone, which is the foundation of your face. Who doesn't want to have a face with a firm foundation?

YOU HAVE DEMYSTIFIED DENTISTRY

You demystified dentistry, and provided solid reasons to think long term. Many people avoid the dentist day by day, month by month, but they don't face the truth of the long-term consequences.

The story about Melanie Greene, your 70-year-old patient with cancer, was touching. If she had come to you even a few months later, it wouldn't have been possible for you to save her upper teeth. Even at 70, a few months can make a world of difference.

Then we ended on a lighter note around looking better, feeling better. Feeling more dynamic, making more money, making more friends.

Janice:
Dating!

Aurora:
Getting a megawatt smile like a Hollywood star! You two are awesome.

So the benefits include everything from self-care to feeling more confident to being more beautiful to being healthier to living longer, all simply by making a habit of seeing your dentist every three months.

You have made quite a contribution to my understanding of my own body. Until now, I didn't have the operator's manual for my mouth. Thank you.

Justene:
(laughs)
You're very welcome.

Aurora:
Thanks for sharing your personal story, too. What an amazing odyssey. It's hard to feel uncomfortable or ashamed sharing anything with you. It's hard to feel anything but gratitude. Your story of attempting to escape, and then ending up in a concentration camp was riveting. As was your "Stranger in a Strange Land" experience arriving in America.

And look at you both now smiling with big beautiful smiles. From such humble beginnings, you are now successful dentists making a difference in the world. You're helping people transform their lives, their health, their beauty, their confidence—and have dazzling smiles, too.

Janice:
Thank you.

Aurora:

You're welcome. Anything else that you would like to add?

Janice:

Our mission statement is to help adults achieve their best possible smile.

Here's my vision for the contribution I'm making as a dentist:

Without my help, these people lack self-confidence and are not fully living up to their full potential. Without my help, these people experience pain, suffering, embarrassment, and compromised health.

But with my help, they instead experience oral health, and also overall health, happiness, vitality, and self-confidence. With good oral health, they add ten or more years to their lives and improve the quality of their later years.

They have a beautiful, healthy smile that lasts well into their later years. I do this to improve their well-being and confidence so

OUR MISSION IS TO HELP ADULTS ACHIEVE THEIR BEST POSSIBLE SMILE that they can, in turn, create positive contributions and make our world a better place.

Aurora:

That's inspiring.

Janice:

It makes me jump out of bed every morning eager to make a difference.

What to Do Next

Aurora:

I'll bet a lot of people are eager to get a healthy, beautiful smile now. What should people do next?

Justene:

Our website is a great place to start: www. APlusFamilyDentistry.com. People can see our office, our team, and the different services that we offer.

Justene:

We love to meet people in person, so people can call and make an appointment to come in and see us in person.

Aurora:

Call 619-265-2467 or visit www. APlusFamilyDentistry.com to schedule a personal consultation. Watch bonus videos and get other free resources online at www.KeysToAHealthySmileAfter40.com.

Janice:

We love to see people in person. Everyone's different. We customize the right dental solution to meet each person's specific needs and goals.

Aurora:

I love that you want to find out what's right for each person. This book provides general guidelines, but these concepts need to be tailored specifically to each patient and their particular situation.

Justene:

My database says that we have had ten thousand people through our doors over the last 15 years, and we haven't seen two people exactly alike.

Aurora:

Visit www.APlusFamilyDentistry.com. Call 619-265-2467 to make an appointment to see Drs. Justene and Janice Doan so that they can give you a beautiful, youthful smile. Go every quarter to take care of your health.

That was very informative and inspiring. Thank you, Justene and Janice.

About the Authors

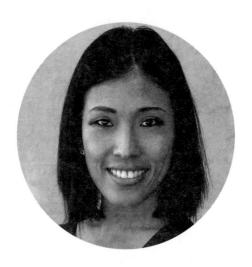

JUSTENE DOAN, DDS

Dr. Justene Doan is a dentist, speaker, and author. Dr. Justene enjoys dentistry because it allows her to pursue her three loves: science, art and helping people.

She opened A+ Family Dentistry in San Diego, California in 2002 with her husband, Dr. Roger Tran. Her sister, Dr. Janice Doan, joined A+ Family Dentistry in 2009.

A highly trained general dentist, Dr. Justene values getting to know each one of her patients. She takes the time to listen atten-tively and explain procedures thoroughly.

Now over 40 herself, she loves helping patients over 40 rejuvenate their smiles and reclaim their health and confidence.

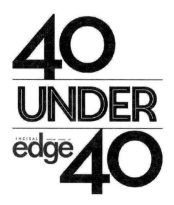

Awards

In 2015, Dr. Justene was selected as one of the 40 Top Dentists Under 40 in the U.S. by "Incisal Edge" magazine. Her sister, Dr. Janice, also received this honor. This honor is given to outstanding dental profession-als who are setting new benchmarks in their industry.

Knowledgeable Implant Dentist

Highly skilled in implant dentistry, Dr. Justene has placed hundreds of implants. Her considerable postgraduate training includes a fellowship program and a year-long surgical externship in implantology. She keeps up-to-date on the latest techniques and procedures in implant dentistry through regular continuing education.

Education

Dr. Justene received her Doctor of Dental Surgery degree from the University of Southern California. A life-long learner, Dr. Justene is dedicated to excellence. Her postgraduate education includes several dental implant training programs, a fellowship program, a year-long surgical externship through the California Implant Institute, dental laser training, a two-year orthodontics curriculum, and more.

Community Service

Dr. Justene contributes to social betterment programs, including anti-drug and human rights campaigns. She also provides pro bono dental services to underserved children. For example, she recently collaborated with TeamSmile and the San Diego Chargers.

About the Authors (cont.)

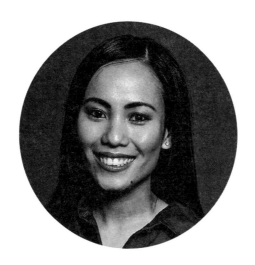

JANICE DOAN, DDS

Dr. Janice Doan practices general and cosmetic dentistry. Her goal is to give her patients a healthy smile that will last a lifetime.

Dr. Janice treats her patients as if they were her own family members. Using excellent communication skills, she explains dental procedures in a simple, clear way.

Dr. Janice and Dr. Justene Doan jointly run A+ Family Dentistry in San Diego, California.

Awards

Dr. Janice was named a "Top 40 Under 40" dentist by "Incisal Edge" magazine, along with her sister Dr. Justene. The 40 under 40 program recognizes innovative and passionate young dental professionals who are raising the standards of dentistry.

Education

Dr. Janice received her Doctor of Dental Science degree from the University of Southern California. Committed to staying on the leading edge, Dr. Janice continues learning. Her postgraduate education covers the latest techniques in dentistry, including dental implants, cosmetic dentistry, endodontics (root canal treatment), Invisalign® and laser dentistry. She has also completed a dental implant fellowship and a surgical externship through the California Implant Institute.

Community Service

Dr. Janice places a high value on giving back to the community and provides pro bono dentistry through numerous volunteer programs, including the USC Mobile Clinic and Special Patients Clinic, and the San Diego Give Kids a Smile Day program, and more.

Visit A+ Family Dentistry

Our team of knowledgeable, friendly doctors and specialists offer comprehensive services, including advanced care, so you can usually have all of your dental needs taken care of in one office.

We will help you create optimal health and a beautiful smile. Make an appointment today!

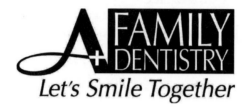

Let's Smile Together

A+ Family Dentistry: San Diego
3780 El Cajon Blvd, Unit #1
San Diego, CA 92105
Phone 619-265-2467

A+ Family Dentistry: Poway
12915 Pomerado Road
Poway, CA 92064
Phone 858-842-5850

www.APlusFamilyDentistry.com